KILLER DIETS

KILLER DIETS

Are Low-Carb Diets High-Risk?

LAURA MUHA

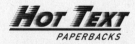

Chamberlain Bros.
a member of Penguin Group (USA) Inc.
New York

CHAMBERLAIN BROS.
Published by the Penguin Group
Penguin Group (USA) Inc., 375 Hudson Street, New York, New York 10014,
USA
Penguin Group (Canada), 10 Alcorn Avenue, Toronto, Ontario, Canada M4V
3B2 (a division of Pearson Penguin Canada Inc.)
Penguin Books Ltd, 80 Strand, London WC2R 0RL, England
Penguin Ireland, 25 St Stephen's Green, Dublin 2, Ireland (a division of
Penguin Books Ltd)
Penguin Group (Australia), 250 Camberwell Road, Camberwell, Victoria
3124, Australia
(a division of Pearson Australia Group Pty Ltd)
Penguin Books India Pvt Ltd, 11 Community Centre, Panchsheel Park, New
Delhi–110 017, India Penguin Group (NZ), cnr Airborne and Rosedale Roads,
Albany, Auckland 1310, New Zealand (a division of Pearson New Zealand
Ltd.)
Penguin Books (South Africa) (Pty) Ltd, 24 Sturdee Avenue, Rosebank,
Johannesburg 2196, South Africa

Penguin Books Ltd, Registered Offices: 80 Strand, London WC2R 0RL,
England

Chamberlain Bros.
a member of Penguin Group (USA) Inc.
375 Hudson Street
New York, NY 10014

While the author has made every effort to provide accurate telephone numbers
and Internet addresses at the time of publication, neither the publisher nor the
author assumes any responsibility for errors, or for changes that occur after
publication.

An application has been submitted to register this book with the Library of
Congress.

ISBN 1-59609-043-X

Printed in the United States of America
10 9 8 7 6 5 4 3 2 1

Book design by Mike Rivilis

To my grandmother, Anna Muha, whose belief in family dinners and good home cooking has influenced me in ways she'll never know.

CONTENTS

Acknowledgments

A book on a subject as phenomenally complicated as this one could not have been written without the assistance of a great many people. I extend my deepest appreciation to all the dieters, physicians, dietitians, and scientists mentioned herein, including Robert Atkins, who graciously spent hours talking to me for a profile several years before his death. On the nonscientific front, I owe a debt of gratitude to Beth Whitehouse, who is not only a top-notch reader (and a top-notch friend) but also generously took over the heavy lifting in other areas of my professional life to free me up as my deadline loomed. Last, there are no words sufficient to express my appreciation to my husband, Beryl Taylor, whose love and support (not to mention his cooking) have fortified me throughout this project, and always.

Introduction

There's a food fight going on in this country, and your health could be at stake. This controversy revolves around some of our most cherished ideas about diet and nutrition:

That fatty foods (such as steak) are bad for our waistlines and our arteries.

That carbohydrates (such as bread, rice, and pasta) make up the foundation of a healthy diet.

Two out of every three people are overweight because we eat way too many calories and watch television all day long.

For nearly a quarter of a century, those ideas, seemingly backed by a slew of scientific studies (not to mention the federal government's Food Pyramid), were so widely accepted that many people attempted to extricate all fat from every part of their diets. We stripped the skin off our chicken (which was broiled, not fried), ordered our fat-free salad dressing on the side, and sloshed skim milk in our coffee when what we really craved was cream. We were aided and abetted in these efforts by the food industry, which flooded the market with hundreds of millions of dollars worth of low- and no-fat versions of our favorite foods: ice cream, potato chips, cookies, etc.

But we kept getting fatter.

By the mid-1990s, 66 percent of people over the age of eighteen weighed more than what was considered healthy, and those under age eighteen weren't doing much better. One in every five children was overweight. Overweight was defined as those whose body mass index—weight adjusted for height—was in the 95th percentile or higher. If the 85th to 95th percentile was also included—a group many pediatricians still considered too heavy—the rate jumped to one in four.

Even more alarming was that the size of our waistlines wasn't only a cosmetic issue. By 2001, an estimated 400,000 people were dying of weight-related problems every year, making obesity-related illnesses second only to tobacco-related illnesses on the list of preventable causes of death. The number of people with weight- and diet-related illnesses, including heart disease, stroke, high blood pressure, type 2 diabetes, arthritis, gallbladder disease—and even some cancers—kept climbing, or (in the case of heart disease) at least didn't decline the way we'd expected it would after we bought into the low-fat message. Even preschoolers were showing evidence of high blood pressure and high cholesterol, and type 2 diabetes—once rarely seen before middle age— began cropping up in children, with enough frequency that doctors could no longer accurately refer to it by its previous name: "adult-onset diabetes." Health-care expenses stemming from overweight and obesity cost $117 billion every year.

It is no wonder, then, that when a series of new studies with completely counterintuitive results began making news a couple years ago, everyone started to pay attention.

In these studies, done at some of the country's leading medical institutions, overweight patients were divided into groups and placed on either a conventional low-fat diet or one in which they were allowed to eat as much fat and protein as they wanted but had to restrict their carbohydrate intake.

The latter approach was based on a controversial diet first popularized during the 1970s and repopularized in the 1990s by the late Robert Atkins,

M.D., a New York cardiologist and author of the best-selling diet book of all time, Dr. Atkins' New Diet Revolution.

Dr. Atkins had long insisted that fat wasn't the dietary villain we were making it out to be. He maintained that the real culprit behind the growing weight problem in America was carbohydrates; if we cut those from our diet, he said, we could eat fat to our heart's content—literally—because of metabolic shifts that would keep fat from building up on the walls of our arteries or settling around our bodies. The idea was viewed by the medical establishment as so ludicrous that until the late 1990s, when so many people were on low-carb diets that doctors could no longer look the other way, nobody had even bothered to study it. After all, didn't we know what the results from eating so much fat would be?

As it turned out, we didn't. To the amazement of just about everyone—except Dr. Atkins's followers—people on the low-carb plan lost more weight on average than those on the conventional diet—at least in the short term—and in many cases, their cholesterol and triglyceride levels improved more. "That was what shocked us and everybody else—that you could eat more fat and have beneficial changes to your cholesterol profile," says William

Yancy, M.D., an obesity specialist and assistant professor of medicine at Duke University Medical Center, one of the lead investigators on two of the initial studies, the first of which was published in 2002.

The new studies were greeted with glee by longtime fans of low-carb diets, and with dismay by nutritionists, many of whom didn't entirely dismiss the findings but worried that they were being oversimplified by the media and that their implications were being misunderstood by a public eager to find a quick solution to its collectively expanding waistline.

Organizations such as the American Dietetic Association and the American Heart Association rushed to point out that years of research showed that diets rich in whole grains, fruits, and vegetables— foods which typically contain high levels of carbohydrates and therefore tend to be limited on low-carb diets—were broadly protective against heart disease, diabetes, and cancer. And they warned that the increased fat and protein taken in by low-carb dieters would not only increase risk of those diseases but also of kidney problems, osteoporosis, liver disease, gout, and many other chronic health problems.

The organizations' predictions were dismissed as scare tactics by many low-carb enthusiasts. However, they in turn were denounced by the pro-carb contingent as irresponsible for rushing to promote the diet when so many serious questions still remained. "You can lose weight on chemotherapy, but that doesn't mean it's good for you," said longtime Atkins critic and low-fat diet advocate Dean Ornish, M.D.

The battle has been raging ever since, its tone sometimes taking on an antagonism more common to election-year politics than dietary discourses. Pro-carb groups have been called everything from the "grease gestapo" to the "vegetarian Taliban" (this last by Atkins's widow, Veronica, during a Dateline NBC interview).

Even New York City Mayor Michael Bloomberg has been dragged into the fray, making national headlines after making an offhand comment that he thought Atkins—who died in 2003 after slipping on an icy sidewalk and striking his head—was "fat" and that his diet was inedible. Unaware that the television cameras were rolling, the mayor also confided that while attending a fundraiser at Atkins's home a few years before the doctor's death, "I took one appetizer and I had to spit it into my napkin."

He later apologized to Veronica Atkins.

At the medical and governmental level, the discussion has been equally heated—so much so that a debate on the subject, sponsored several years ago by the U.S. Department of Agriculture, threatened at times to degenerate into a sniping match between diet doctors. At the debate's end, it was clear that it's sometimes difficult to separate the science of food from the personalities and politics involved.

The seemingly endless parade of contradictory headlines—some appearing within weeks of one another—has confused things even further:

AT LAST, REAL PROOF THAT THE ATKINS DIET WORKS

DESPITE HYPE, HIGH-FAT ATKINS DIET DOESN'T TRIM WEIGHT

LOW-CARB DIETERS KNEW IT ALL ALONG: IN TWO RECENT STUDIES ATKINS-STYLE REGIMEN BROUGHT FASTER RESULTS

STUDIES SAY ATKINS DIET A SHORT-TERM FIX

IS IT OVER FOR ATKINS?

It's unlikely that the low-carb craze is over. In the past two years, what was once viewed as a fringe movement has become a trend that shows no sign of losing force anytime soon. In surveys, 44 percent of people now say they're trying to limit their carbohydrate intake in some way, and one of every six households includes someone on a full-fledged low-carb diet. Six out of the top fifteen books on The New York Times bestseller list on one week in late 2004 were related to low-carb diets. The one that started it all—Dr. Atkins' New Diet Revolution— was only recently bumped from that list after a run that had been virtually uninterrupted since 1997. The list of stars who have reportedly tried low-carb diets reads like a who's who in Hollywood: Jennifer Aniston, Brad Pitt, Matt LeBlanc, Matthew Perry, Whoopi Goldberg, Renée Zellweger, Geri Halliwell, Bette Midler, Minnie Driver, and Stevie Nicks, to name just a few.

The food industry has jumped on the bandwagon, too, seeming to respond to the low-carb craze the way it did for the low-fat trend a decade ago. In the first six months of 2004, the industry pumped millions of dollars worth of new low-carb products into the marketplace: low-carb ice cream, donuts, beer, pasta, pancake mixes, cereal, cookies, and bread.

In restaurants, "heart-friendly" low-fat entrees are being pushed off menus by "carb friendly" choices. And the low-carb frenzy has sliced so deeply into the bakery business that an industry group called the Bread Leadership Council called a "bread summit" to stimulate "meaningful discussion around key nutrition issues surrounding bread." Another industry group, The North American Millers' Association, reported that annual flour consumption dropped from 147 pounds per person in 1997 to 137 pounds in 2002.

An even stronger indication that low-carb diets are here to stay, however, may be the fact that some of the country's most respected physicians have come to conditionally accept the possibility that the diets may be successful. "We can no longer dismiss very-low-carbohydrate diets," Walter Willett, M.D., wrote last year in an editorial published in The Annals of Internal Medicine. Since Willett is chairman of the nutrition department at Harvard's prestigious School of Public Health, this quote was widely repeated in newspapers, as well as low-carb-related Internet sites, where it was held up as "proof" that low-carb diets are safe and effective.

Why, then, do many dietitians and doctors— including Willett—remain so concerned? Are they, as many low-carb fans seem to think, just a bunch of dissenters, clinging to outdated ideas because they're too stubborn to admit they were wrong? Or is it something more than that?

While all the name-calling and finger-pointing that has been going on have made for entertaining reading, one of the things the doctors haven't provided is context—something desperately needed by those of us trying to sort through the confusion in order to make informed health decisions. Of course, putting a subject as complex as nutrition into context is no simple task, since it must take into account so many things: history, politics, personalities, big business, genetics, biochemistry, environment, and the lifestyle choices of individuals, not to mention the nuances of science and the difficulty of communicating those nuances to members of the public, who tend to see the results of a study and think they "prove" something. Scientists, on the other hand, are aware that the weight of evidence can flip-flop almost overnight. Remember all the studies that seemed to "prove" that hormone-replacement therapy prevented heart disease—until a more definitive study showed that it might in some cases actually cause it?

"There are many strong things being said

without any information, without any data, to back them up," says Willett. "And that includes most of the official dietary recommendations from government groups, from professional organizations, many nutritionists, as well as the people who write popular diet books."

The bottom line is that while the new studies do suggest that low-carb diets may play an important role in helping some people lose weight, there remains a great deal we don't know about how low-carb diets will affect us over a period of time longer than the six months to a year that dieters have so far been studied.

Diane Stadler, Ph.D., a biochemical nutrition specialist and research assistant professor at Oregon Health & Science University, says she thinks low-carb diets can be "a powerful tool" for weight loss, but not one that people ought to consider using lightly. "I think people are being pretty cavalier about this," she says. "Not intentionally—but I don't think they perceive that there's any risk. And I'm not sure we're at the point where we can say there's no risk—or even that there's very little risk. I think that for some people, there might be significant risk."

But until we have many more years worth of studies, we won't really know who's at risk—or exactly what they're at risk of. Much of what's being said about low-carb diets—by low-carbers and pro-carbers alike—are projections based on information extrapolated from nutrition studies that weren't specifically looking at low-carb diets. As history has shown again and again, extrapolation can be dangerous. "We have to try to stick to what we know and not guess what we believe will happen," says Yancy.

But that doesn't mean, he adds, that no one should consider going on a low-carb diet until all the results are in; most of us can't afford to wait that long to do something about the excess pounds we're lugging around. It does mean, however, that we shouldn't ditch the dinner rolls and pour a ladle full of béarnaise sauce over that slab of prime rib before we educate ourselves about the potential risks and benefits involved, and consider all of our options.

After all, our health is at stake.

1.

Low-Carb vs. Low-Fat:
The Battle Begins

I f it wasn't for one ID card photograph, today's dietary debate might be very different.

It was 1963, and Robert C. Atkins, M.D., was a young cardiologist building a private practice in New York City. He had just accepted a part-time consulting position at AT&T. When his picture was taken for the company identification card, he was horrified at what he saw. "I just kept looking at that and saying, 'My God, I have three chins!' " he would recall in an interview years later.

It was the kind of moment that many of us have had at one point or another—when we're forced to face the fact that the image we hold of ourselves in our head no longer matches the image reflected back in the mirror. Most people deal with it by resolving to immediately go on a diet and then hastily push it out of their minds. Or, if they are really determined, by temporarily cutting back on the donuts and desserts until they lose a few pounds.

But for Atkins, the consequences of that moment would affect far more than the number on his bathroom scale. Although he couldn't have known it at the time, his concerns over that ID card photo were the first step toward what nearly four decades later would blow up into one of the most bitter scientific controversies of the century—one that is now being played out not only in laboratories and on the pages of medical journals but in headlines and at dinner tables across the country.

This debate, centered on what's made us all so fat and the best way to fix it, would have eventually happened without Dr. Atkins. But there's little doubt that his single-minded devotion to the cause kept the idea alive even when almost everyone else seemed to be on the other side of the argument. With his alternately charming and abrasive personality—this is a man who once told a dietitian on national TV that if her mind were as broad as her hips, she might learn something—it's no wonder the spotlight kept coming back to him. That would not only help drive the debate but in the process would turn Atkins's once-struggling medical practice into a multimillion-dollar business empire that many experts agree is changing the American dietary landscape.

In 1963, however, all this controversy lay many years in the future. In those days, Atkins was, as he put it, "as mainstream as you could be"—just another thirtysomething New Yorker trying to figure out what to do about the spare tire around his middle. It was a new scenario for the young cardiologist, who'd never had a weight problem while growing up in Dayton, Ohio; in fact, just the opposite was true. "When I got out of high school, I was six feet tall and weighed only 135 pounds," he wrote in 1972. "I was the skinniest kid on the block."

Although Atkins had eaten his way to a more normal weight in college, it wasn't until he graduated from Cornell University's medical school in 1955 that he really began packing on the pounds—so many of them that by the time that ID-card photo was taken eight years later, the man who'd once been the skinniest kid on the block weighed well over 200 pounds. That was almost thirty pounds more than he wanted to weigh—but not just for the sake of his health. "I [was] a bachelor with an incredible interest in running around," he recalled with a chuckle. "I said, 'No one's going to be interested in me!'"

Still, Atkins had, as he put it, "one hell of an appetite," and the thought of dieting, which he equated with going hungry, depressed him. "I knew about diets," he wrote. "But the trouble was they all told me to stop when I had eaten seven or eight ounces of my steak. That's only half a portion. I knew from experience that halfway through a steak, I was hungrier than when I sat down. I knew that I could never follow a low-calorie diet for even one day."

So Atkins began looking through medical literature, searching for articles on alternative ways to lose weight that might give him, as he put it, "some sort of clue as to what I could do for myself." He soon stumbled across a study in a medical journal on fasting, which in the 1960s was a popular way to lose a few pounds. He was fascinated to learn that subjects described a sharp decrease in hunger after the first couple days of not eating. "That stunned me," he wrote. "Incredible that I could find myself not hungry after going without food for forty-eight hours. How could that possibly be? That defied logic. I wanted to know why."

The researchers who'd written the article attributed the loss of hunger to the presence of ketones in the blood. These ketones—essentially organic compounds, microscopic fragments of carbon—are created when the body runs out of carbohydrates, and instead turns to burning its fat reserves as fuel. "In every case, there was a relationship between [high blood levels of ketones] and loss of appetite," the researchers wrote.

Ketogenic diets—that is, diets that produced high levels of ketones—weren't a new concept. Physicians at the Mayo Clinic had been using them since the 1920s to treat seizures in children who had epilepsy, a purpose for which such diets are still used today. The diet wasn't one most people would choose to go on—children were literally subsisting on fatty foods such as sausages, washed down with heavy cream— but it often worked, not only bringing the seizures under control but sometimes also permanently eliminating them, so that the children could resume eating normal foods. However, ketogenic diets hadn't really been discussed in reference to weight loss, and while inducing ketosis by fasting obviously wasn't the solution for Atkins, he did recognize that it might be a piece of a much larger dietary puzzle.

So he kept plowing through the literature, and before long he came across the work of a physician named Alfred W. Pennington. Pennington was hired by the DuPont Company in the 1940s to determine why so many employees were having trouble losing weight. Theorizing that the problem lay not with their caloric intake but with their metabolism, Pennington put twenty of the employees on a 3,000-calorie-a-day diet that allowed them to eat plenty of fat and protein, but virtually no sugar and starch. Dieters lost an average of twenty-two pounds each in three and a half months, and many reduced their blood pressure as well. Even more exciting to Atkins was the fact that the dieters said they never felt hungry on the diet.

Not long afterward, he was reading one medical journal and the final piece of the puzzle fell into place. A study by Atlanta researchers Walter Lyons Bloom and Gordon Azar reported that patients didn't have to stop eating altogether to achieve ketosis; simply cutting out carbohydrates while continuing to eat foods such as meat and salad seemed to have the same effect. "Bloom and Azar's paper convinced me to go on the only diet I've ever been on," Atkins would later say.

Since ketones were so essential to his new diet, Atkins knew he'd need a way to monitor their presence. If ketones were in the blood, they would also be present in urine, and could be detected using a specific tablet that measures ketones and turned purple when they were present. Atkins got these tablets, which were readily available in drugstores, swore off bread and potatoes, and went grocery shopping.

At first Atkins eliminated all carbohydrates from his diet. But he soon discovered that the ketone-test tablet would turn purple—meaning that his body was continuing to burn fat—even if he ate small quantities of carbohydrates. "That meant some vegetables, sometimes melon, big, fresh strawberries smothered in whipped cream . . . an occasional Scotch and water before dinner," he wrote. "I found as time went on that I could have thirty-five to forty grams of carbohydrates a day and still lose, without hunger."

When Atkins went on his experimental diet, he expected to lose a few pounds every month. Instead, he lost twenty-five pounds in the first six weeks, even though he was eating constantly, going home from the hospital three times a day to fill himself up. "It was so exciting—it was almost as if the more you ate, the more you lost," he recalled in an interview years later. Equally exciting, he said, was that he went from needing eight or nine hours of sleep a night to needing only five and a half. "Thinking back on that time, I didn't realize how sleepy, tired, and lazy I had always been until I went on my diet," he wrote. "It was only after I had been on the diet that I noticed the improvement and suddenly realized that I really hadn't been feeling up to par."

Astonished and delighted by his success, Atkins convinced his colleagues in the medical department at AT&T to let him put sixty-five overweight members of the company's junior-executive program on the diet the following year to see if it would work for them. "My mind was blown by the fact that every single one of them got down to their goal weight," he recalled years later. "Talk about beginner's luck— it would be like Tiger Woods shooting fifty-four the first time playing golf!"

Not one to keep such success to himself, Atkins went to work refining the diet to make it accessible to a larger number of people. Word spread, and in 1965 he was invited to appear on The Tonight Show to talk about it. A magazine article appeared the following year, and that got the attention of a book publisher.

Dr. Atkins' Diet Revolution was published in 1972 and became an immediate hit with the public, remaining on The New York Times bestseller list for 100 straight weeks. The medical community was much less enthusiastic. In a review, the American Medical Association blasted Atkins as "naïve" and his diet as "biochemically incorrect," "grossly unbalanced," and "potentially dangerous."

Furious, he resigned from the AMA—less because of the scathing review itself, he said later, than because when he checked the citations to see which studies the authors had used to support their opinions, he couldn't find any evidence that they'd even looked at the studies on which he'd based his diet. "What this proved to me was that the leaders of medicine were intellectually dishonest," Atkins recalled, still sounding indignant about it thirty years later. "I never considered myself a fighter, but that turned me into a fighter. I took a pledge that I was going to prove them wrong, and my whole life has been dedicated to that."

Part of the reason for the clash—which was nothing compared to the full-scale nutrition war that would break out three decades later—was that the diet Atkins was promoting flew in the face of years of widely accepted scientific data.

By World War II, heart disease had become the leading killer of Americans (a dubious distinction that it continues to hold today). Food, which had been largely a do-it-yourself proposition when our great-great-grandparents were growing up, was becoming a commodity. The food industry was growing steadily—first to provision the troops during the war, and later to take advantage of an increase in disposable income as well as the public's desire for more leisure time in the postwar era.

Into this changing picture stepped a Minnesota biologist and epidemiologist by the name of Ancel Keys, who would later say that he noticed the heart-disease trend in the obituary pages of the newspaper.

Keys suspected that diet played a role in cardiovascular disease for two reasons: First, its incidence in Europe had fallen sharply during World War II, when the availability of food—particularly meat and dairy products—was restricted. Second, studies done on rabbits by Russian researchers had shown that blood levels of cholesterol were directly linked to the amounts of fat in the diet the animals were fed.

With this in mind, Keys embarked on a series of studies that would make him a household name in his era and still famous among scientists a halfcentury later.

In one study—which would be considered unethical today, but in that day wasn't uncommon—Keys and his associates tinkered with the diets of patients in state mental hospitals, varying the proportion of fats and carbohydrates they were eating, particularly looking at the impact of butter, corn oil, olive oil, and vegetable shortening on their cholesterol levels. In another, they signed up 283 men living in Minneapolis and St. Paul for a long-term study in which they tracked what was in the men's diets and how many of them developed heart disease as a result.

They found that the men's likelihood of having a heart attack was closely correlated with blood pressure, smoking habits, and cholesterol levels, and that the men's cholesterol levels seemed to depend on how much saturated fat they were eating.

Unquestionably, Keys's most famous study was known as the Seven Countries Study, which tracked the diets of men living in seven industrialized nations—Finland, Greece, Yugoslavia, Italy, the Netherlands, Japan, and the United States—and found that in countries where people ate less fat, there were lower rates of heart disease.

In 1959, eager to get the public to break what he called "the North American habit for making the stomach the garbage disposal unit for a long list of harmful foods," Keys published one of the first low-fat cookbooks, Eat Well and Stay Well. In it, he laid out his prescription for good health, which even today remains the cornerstone of most disease-prevention advice, regardless of whether the person who dispenses it advocates a pro- or low-carb approach: maintain a healthy weight; restrict consumption of saturated fats; eat plenty of vegetables, fruit, and products made from skim milk (low-carb proponents say you should drink whole milk); avoid too much sugar and salt; quit smoking; and get plenty of exercise. Keys's findings paralleled those of a series of studies sponsored by the American Heart Association in the 1950s, and his advice was reiterated by the organization, which around that time began urging Americans to get no more than 35 percent of their calories from fat (and no more than 10 percent from saturated fat).

Public awareness built slowly in the 1960s. When Atkins's book came out in 1972, the low-fat message wasn't yet in fully accepted, but was starting to be recognized. "Cholesterol" had become a buzzword, even among the less-than-health conscious, and just about everyone seemed to be counting calories. Then, in the mid-1970s, a congressional committee, the Select Committee on Nutrition and Human Needs, held a series of hearings looking at the impact of diet on health—specifically heart disease, obesity and diabetes. The result was a 1977 report titled

"Dietary Goals for the United States," which recommended that Americans increase their carbohydrate consumption but decrease their intake of fat, cholesterol, sugar, and salt.

Cattle and dairy farmers, sensing that these recommendations could have catastrophic consequences for their industries, went ballistic, and so did producers of sugar and eggs. This marked the beginning of a pattern of industry intervening with nutrition advice issued by the federal government. After heavy lobbying, the congressional commission held another series of hearings and came out with a new report that replaced their original recommendation to "reduce consumption of meat" with a phrase encouraging Americans to "choose meats, poultry, and fish which will reduce saturated fat intake."

The report helped to cement the low-fat message in the public's mind, and institutionalized it among the organizations that issued dietary advice, not only non-rofit groups such as the American Heart Association but also the U.S. government, which began issuing national health guidelines recommending that Americans lower their fat intake. The food industry, seizing the opportunity, jumped in and began cranking out low-fat foods that

Americans started immediately buying.

The resulting low-fat trend swept Atkins and his "eat fat, not carbs" message from the spotlight for two decades. He still had a steady stream of loyal followers who believed in his diet, but when it came to the national dietary debate, Atkins spent much of the next quarter-century on the sidelines.

"The low-fat diet was the first really national nutritional experiment that we've ever had, and it's failed," says Michael Eades, M.D., who with his wife, Mary Dan Eades, M.D., is coauthor of *Protein Power*.

Not everyone agrees with him—or at least agrees that the failure was due to the low-fat message itself. "I think it was in part a phenomenon of the food industry picking up on something that could be exploited for commercial benefit," says Ruth Kava, Ph.D., nutrition director for the American Council on Science and Health, a nonprofit consumer-education group.

Manufacturers not only cranked out low-fat products but also marketed them in such a way that implied that they were healthier than their higher-fat counterparts. And the public bought right into it. Before long, the message that had started out as "cut some of the fat from your diet" became "fat makes you fat." And from there it was a quick jump to "avoid fat and you won't get fat." As way too many of us learned the hard way, that is not the truth.

"The mantra from the medical profession was 'eat less fat'—and clearly what that did was give people license to eat unlimited quantities of carbohydrates, which was insanity," says Linda Stern, M.D., a clinical assistant professor of medicine with the University of Pennsylvania Health System and author of two recent low-carb studies.

Because low-fat eating was the main concern, we didn't even realize how many more carbs we were eating, says Kava. Portion sizes were growing subtly larger, and as manufacturers pulled fat from products, they replaced it with high-fructose corn syrup. In fact, while some people say we're eating more carbs than we used to, that's true only in terms of the number of carbohydrate calories we're consuming. The basic carb-fat-protein ratio of most Americans' diets has essentially stayed the same as it was in the years prior to the obesity epidemic, says Kava. "We increased the denominator instead of decreasing the numerator," she explains.

In the end, though, it didn't matter to most of us why the low-fat message failed; the point was that weight wasn't being lost, and we were frustrated.

After all, we'd done what everyone from the federal government to the nutrition experts told us to do: We'd trimmed fat, chosen lean meats and low-fat sour cream, switched from bacon and eggs to bagels—so why were we gaining weight? In frustration, we began turning our backs on low-fat foods and returning to cheeseburgers—hold the bun—even as the mainstream medical establishment pleaded with us to come to our senses. In the 1990s, America's growing waistline propelled Dr. Atkins directly to the center of a new and increasingly bitter controversy.

This time, however, Atkins had company. When a revised edition of *Dr. Atkins' New Diet Revolution* was published in 1992, it didn't take long before it was joined on bookshelves by familiar titles such as *The Zone*, *Protein Power*, *Sugar Busters!*, *The Carbohydrate Addict's Diet*, *Suzanne Somers' Eat Great, Lose Weight*, *The Paleo Diet* and *Neanderthin* (both of which outlined the meat-based diet of our caveman ancestors), and, in 2003, the phenomenally popular *South Beach Diet*. Although the diets all had slightly different strategies, all were rooted in the same basic premise: It's not fat that's made us fat, it's carbs.

Likes it or not, low-carb diets looked as though they were here to stay.

A Brief History of the Low-Carb Diet

Although Robert Atkins is often credited with "discovering" low-carb dieting, the concept actually predated him by nearly 140 years. Here's a brief history of the low-carb diet.

1825: In his book *The Physiology of Taste*, French lawyer and gastronome Jeane Anthelme Brillate-Savarin declares that "a more or less rigid abstinence from everything that is starchy or floury will lead to the lessening of weight" and prescribes what may well have been the first low-carb diet: "[S]hun anything made with flour, no matter in what form it hides; do you not still have the roast, the salad, the leafy vegetables?"

1860s: London carpenter William Banting, who sometimes served as an undertaker to the rich and famous, self-publishes a pamphlet titled "Letter on Corpulence," which he sells for a shilling. In it, he describes how he lost fifty pounds by eliminating bread, milk, sugar, and potatoes, and outlines his new diet: mutton, kidneys or broiled fish for breakfast; herring, eels, or poultry and vegetables for lunch; meat or fish for supper. (He also confesses to one starchy vice: "Being fond of green peas, I take them daily in the season, and I gain 2 or 3 lbs in weight as well as some little in bulk, but I soon lose both when [the pea] season is over.") His diet became so popular that by 1869, more than 63,000 copies had been sold, and "banting" became slang for dieting—a word that is still used in Britain today.

1888: Chicago physician James H. Salisbury encourages patients to stop eating vegetables, starches, and fruits because, he says, they cause the stomach to become "flabby and baggy" and give off toxins that lead to a wide range of diseases, including arthrosclerosis, tuberculosis, and gout. He prescribes instead a diet consisting of "the muscle pulp of lean beef made into cakes and broiled," taken three times a day with hot water to keep the system flushed out. (A somewhat tastier version of this recipe, sans the hot-water chaser, survives today in the form of Salisbury steak.)

1920s: Physicians at the Mayo Clinic begin using restricted-carbohydrate diets to treat seizures in epilepsy patients.

1940s: Dr. Alfred W. Pennington puts twenty DuPont employees on a 3,000-calorie low-carb diet. They lose an average of twenty-two pounds each in three and a half months.

1963: Using himself as a guinea pig, Atkins tests the first version of what will become his famous diet. A magazine article about it sends patients flocking to his New York office.

1967: New York physician Irwin Stillman publishes *The Doctor's Quick Weight-Loss Diet*, which virtually forbids both carbs and fat.

1972: *Dr. Atkins' Diet Revolution* is published and becomes an instantaneous hit, spending 100 weeks on the New York Times bestseller list.

Other Low-Carb Diets

Although the Atkins diet is probably the most famous low-carb plan, it's far from the only one. Here are just a few others:

- **Stillman Diet**: This plan was developed in the 1960s by Irwin Stillman, a New York physician who believed eating protein almost exclusively was the key to losing weight, because protein is so molecularly complex that the body must expend large amounts of energy to metabolize it. The diet contains almost no carbs and very little fat. The only foods allowed are lean meats, chicken, turkey, fish, eggs, cottage cheese, broth, and artificially sweetened gelatin. The diet has two phases—the "Quick Weight Loss" phase and a "Stay Slim" phase; the latter includes slightly larger quantities of fats and carbs than the former. Dr. Stillman died of a heart attack at the height of his diet's popularity.

- **The Scarsdale Diet**: Developed in the 1970s by Scarsdale, New York, cardiologist Herman Tarnower, M.D., this diet consists mostly of lean protein, fruits, and vegetables. It not only limits dieters to 700 largely carb-free calories per day but also includes menus, which dieters are supposed to follow exactly. Breakfast, for instance, must consist of grapefruit and a slice of high-protein bread without butter. Lunch consists of cold cuts and tomatoes, and dinner is fish or shellfish, salad, another slice of high-protein bread, and grapefruit. The only snacks allowed are carrots and celery. Dr. Tarnower said followers would lose about a pound a day for the week to two weeks they were supposed to be on the diet. Dr. Tarnower went from fame to infamy in 1980 when his girlfriend, in a rage because he had taken up with a younger woman, shot and killed him.

- **The Zone:** Followers of this diet are encouraged to get 40 percent of their calories from carbs, 30 percent from protein, and 30 percent from fat—not just over the course of the day but with each meal and snack. The combination, according to Zone founder Barry Sears, Ph.D., keeps insulin levels in the ideal range, warding off both hunger and weight gain. While many dietitians consider The Zone to be a high-fat, low-carb diet because the percentage of carbs it includes is fewer than the 55 to 60 percent recommended by the American Heart Association, Sears doesn't think of it that way. "The Zone Diet advises moderation in all things—protein, carbs, and fats," Sears writes on his website. Sears worked at MIT before founding his own lab. His specialty is the role of hormones in drug delivery systems.

- **Protein Power:** This diet was developed by Michael and Mary Dan Eades, physicians practicing in Little Rock, Arkansas. The authors believe insulin is responsible for many people's weight problems, and their diet is aimed at helping dieters control their level of that hormone. In its induction phase, the diet starts out with thirty to forty grams of carbohydrates and a set amount of protein, which is specific to the individual dieter and determined by body measurements. The rest of the calories come from fat, although the authors emphasize healthy, unsaturated fats. As the dieter loses weight, he or she adjusts the carbohydrate and protein ratios accordingly. The Eadeses developed the diet based on a study of what our caveman ancestors ate.

- **Sugar Busters!:** Developed by three respected physicians from New Orleans, this diet operates on the premise that sugar is toxic to our systems, because it makes us produce too much insulin. Like most other low-carb diets, Sugar Busters! restricts carbohydrates, and those carbs that are permitted are largely whole grains and fruits. The authors say that dieters who follow their recommendations will end up eating about 40 percent of their calories from carbohydrates, 30 percent from fat, and 30 percent from protein.

• **The South Beach Diet:** The newest addition to the low-carb diet category, the South Beach plan was developed by Miami cardiologist Arthur Agatston. It was an immediate bestseller when published in 2003. It is sometimes referred to as "Atkins lite," because it emphasizes lean meats, whole grains and healthier fats, for which it gets generally good reviews from many dietitians. Aside from the induction phase, which severely restricts carbohydrates, it generally gets good reviews from many mainstream nutrition experts. President Clinton lost a large amount of weight on this diet, but it received some negative press when the former president underwent emergency bypass surgery in 2004.

2.

An Introduction to Metabolism

The parts of food that contain calories are called "macronutrients," and there are only three of them: protein, fat and carbohydrates. Macronutrients are to our bodies what gas is to our car—in other words, we burn them for fuel.

For years, health experts have recommended that we get 45 to 65 percent of our calories from carbohydrates, 20 to 35 percent from fat, and 10 to 35 percent from protein—a balance that they say promotes optimal health.

But low-carb advocates have long argued that those proportions are skewed. Far from promoting health, they say, eating such a carb-heavy diet sets off a metabolic chain reaction that causes us to put on weight and may lead to a host of other chronic diseases as well. That, however, is one of the few things on which they agree.

"The term 'low-carb' actually refers to a whole continuum or spectrum of diets," explains Linda Stern, M.D., of the University of Pennsylvania Health System. "So when people say 'What are low-carb diets like; are they healthy?' you have to define your terms, or you may not wind up talking about the same thing."

Dieters on the Atkins plan, for instance, are told to start out by eating no more than twenty grams of carbohydrates per day in the induction phase of the plan—meaning that no more than 1 percent of the calories on a 2,000-calorie-a-day diet should come from carbohydrates. As dieters near their goal weight, they begin adding carbs back into their meals but rarely get above a total of 100 grams a day, or 5 percent of their caloric intake. The rest of what they're consuming is fat and protein, although the proportions depend to some degree on which foods the dieter selects—choosing steak over chicken, for instance, or cheese over fish.

On The Zone Diet, on the other hand, the ratio of carbs to fat and protein is fixed, and it's quite different from the ratio consumed by Atkins dieters, with 40 percent of calories coming from carbs, 30 percent from protein, and 30 percent from fat. Dieters are supposed to stick to that ratio—not just over the course of the day, but each time they eat a meal or snack.

On Protein Power, meanwhile, dieters start out with forty grams of carbohydrates during the induction phase—which works out to be about 10 percent of the total calories for the average person—and goes up from there as dieters move through the three phases of the program.

The problem with such diets in many experts' minds isn't necessarily the lack of carbs—it's the fact that when you eliminate them, you have to replace them with something, and there are only two other choices. "Inevitably, you're going to be eating more fat and possibly more protein as well," explains Harvard's Walter Willett, M.D. That's a potential problem, because eating large quantities of fat—namely saturated fat—and/or protein have been implicated in the development or progression of some chronic diseases.

In order to understand the theory behind low-carb diets, it helps to know a little about basic metabolism.

Carbohydrates

Found almost exclusively in foods that come from plants, carbs are our body's favorite source of fuel, and it will burn them before it burns either fat or protein.

There are two basic types of carbs: simple and complex. If you asked a molecular biologist the difference, he or she would probably go into a long explanation about the structure of the molecules that make up each of them and the amount of effort your body has to put into metabolizing them. But, generally speaking, it comes down to this: Simple carbs are sugars. Complex carbs are starches, which your body breaks down into sugars.

Now let's talk about what happens when you eat carbohydrates. To you, that thing on the end of your fork might look like a spoonful of mashed potato or a mound of rice. But to your body, it's chock-full of nutrients.

When you put a carb into your mouth, the enzymes in your saliva go to work on it, starting to unwrap it chemically. It then moves in this half-opened state along your digestive system, straight through your stomach and into your small intestine, where enzymes produced by your pancreas break it down the rest of the way. What started life at the upper end of your digestive system as a spoonful of potatoes has now been reduced to a bunch of sugars that easily pass through your intestinal wall into your bloodstream, ready to be used as energy by the cells in many of your body's systems. The problem is that the two can't get together on their own – they need a matchmaker to set them up. So your ever-busy pancreas steps up to the plate and starts cranking out insulin, a hormone that sends out a chemical message to let the cells know there's glucose in the neighborhood. The cells respond by opening up and letting the glucose inside. If there's extra, it's stored as glycogen in the muscles and liver.

Protein

Protein is often referred to as the body's building block, and with good reason. Your brain, your skin, your muscles, your blood cells, and even your fingernails are all made of it. In fact, if you sucked all the water out of your body, three quarters of everything that was left would be protein.

While carbohydrates are made of sugars, proteins are made up of organic compounds called amino acids. If you were to look at them under a microscope, they'd look like long, twisted chains, with each link consisting of an amino acid. Although we tend to equate protein with meat and dairy products, there actually are plenty of plant foods—including beans, grains, and nuts—that are full of protein.

While your body uses carbohydrates as fuel, it

mostly uses protein (or, more accurately, the amino acids that form protein) to repair and rebuild itself. It also uses them in the manufacture of antibodies, enzymes, and hormones.

There are twenty different amino acids that your body needs in order to function. It can make about half of them itself, but the only way you can get the rest is from the protein in your diet. And because your body can't store amino acids the way it can store excess carbohydrates or fats, you have to get them by eating a little bit of protein almost every day. The key words here are "a little bit"—the amount of protein you body needs to get by is about fifty grams if you're an average-sized woman (about the amount contained in a hamburger) and sixty grams if you're an average-sized man. Most Americans—and particularly those on low-carb diets—get a lot more than that, though, which can have some negative consequences.

When you bite into a burger (or a piece of chicken, fish, or tofu), you set off a complex process that begins not in your mouth, as it does for carbohydrates, but in your stomach, where the digestive enzymes begin unraveling the chemical bonds that bind the amino acids together. From there, the amino acids move to your intestine, where more enzymes complete the process. Finally, the amino acids move into your bloodstream, where they, like the glucose from the carbohydrates you've eaten, will be taken up by cells and used for everything from manufacturing hormones to making the neurochemicals that keep your brain functioning, to rebuilding muscle and tissue. Since your body can't store amino acids, it converts them into by-products that you excrete via your urine.

Fat

In the past ten or fifteen years, fat has gotten a bad reputation. Although it's true that it has more than twice as many calories per gram as protein or carbohydrates, that doesn't mean it's all bad for you. In fact, your body needs at least some fat to function. Fat is essential to blood clotting, hormone production, and muscle function. Your cell membranes are made of the stuff, and so are the sheaths around your nerves. Fat also forms a protective cushion around many of your organs. Your body wouldn't be able to absorb vitamins A, D, E or K without fat—and let's not forget that food wouldn't taste nearly as good without fat.

When it comes to breaking down fat, your body faces special problems. Fat isn't soluble in water, so when you eat that juicy slice of beef tenderloin, all the fat globules that make it so nice and tender pass virtually untouched from your mouth straight through your stomach and into your intestines. There, special salts secreted by your gallbladder emulsify it, breaking it into tiny droplets in much the same way that dish detergent breaks down greasy residue on a dinner plate. Your pancreas—a digestive workhorse—then gets into the act, producing more enzymes to break it down further into glycerol (which is essentially a sugar) and fatty acids, which can be either saturated or unsaturated.

Because fats aren't water-soluble, if they move into your bloodstream in their original form, they would coagulate into one big, artery-clogging mass. To prevent this, special cells in the walls of your intestines repackage them into bundles of molecules called chylomicrons, which have triglycerides at their core and a water-soluble exterior. After a couple more complicated steps, they wind up in your bloodstream alongside the glucose and the amino acids.

Your fat cells, which are distributed throughout your body, and are especially concentrated in places such as your abdomen, thighs, and buttocks, serve certain metabolic functions. They serve as little storage lockers for triglycerides, expanding and contracting according to the amount of fat your body is telling them to store. And how does your body do that? Insulin.

Insulin not only connects glucose and your cells, it also lets your fat cells know that there are some triglycerides floating around with no place to go, because they haven't been needed as fuel just yet. So your fat cells kick into gear and start packing them away, just in case you are to need them later.

Unfortunately, many of us never need them later, because there is always plenty of glucose available in our bloodstreams for us to burn. And we since we eat so often and so much in this country, no sooner do we run through the glucose from one meal than we refuel with a snack or another meal.

Which brings us to the theory behind low-carb diets.

If you run out of glucose and fail to supply your body with more—which is what happens when you go on a low-carb diet—your body first turns to whatever it has stashed away (as glycogen) in your liver and muscles. But you'll run out of that in only a day, and when you do, your body will throw a metabolic switch and start burning its second-choice fuel: fat.

On the rare instances when neither is available,

as is the case if someone fasts to the point of starvation, it will burn the only fuel it has left—protein—literally eating away at its own muscles and, as its very last resort, the organs of the body.

To some degree, this happens on most low-carb diets, because while you don't need to *eat* carbohydrates for your body to function, you do need to make them, and the body does this by breaking down muscle tissue, says Joanne Lupton, Ph.D., who holds the William W. Allen Endowed Chair in Nutrition at Texas A&M University.

Lupton recently spent two years sifting through studies on protein, fat and carbohydrates as head of a panel charged with developing something called "dietary reference intakes" for the Institute of Medicine. DRIs are guidelines that are used as, among other things, a basis for the recommended dietary allowances that appear on nutrition labels. To come up with the DRIs, Lupton's committee had to figure out—based on the best science available—the minimum and maximum levels of each macronutrient needed to both prevent nutritional deficiencies and decrease the risk of developing chronic diseases such as osteoporosis, cancer, and cardiovascular disease.

After reviewing all the literature, panel members

concluded that regardless of age or sex, we should all be getting at *least* 130 grams of carbohydrate every day—an amount they determined by looking at how much the brain requires in order to function. Researchers have actually calculated this by feeding glucose into the brain and measuring how much it uses.

But if you don't eat enough carbs to supply your brain with that quantity, it does have another option: It can switch over to burning ketones, the acidic by-products produced when we burn fat, says Lupton.

But not all body systems can do that. Your red blood cells and some of the cells in your eyes, for instance, can only function on glucose. And your body can't get glucose from burning fat. "So if you were on a diet that called for twenty grams of carbohydrate a day, you would break down your own body protein to make carbohydrates out of that," Lupton says. "Because even though you don't have a dietary carbohydrate requirement, you have an absolute requirement for glucose in your body."

And while 130 grams is the absolute minimum that committee members believe we need, the level that they recommend we get is a lot higher—between 45 and 65 percent of our total calories.

However, when you cut so many carbs that your body has to switch over and primarily burn fat, you may enter a state called ketosis—that the level of ketones in your blood and urine is high enough to be measurable. You also give off ketones in your breath, which is why some people complain of bad breath when they go on a low-carb diet. (In fact, what they smell is acetone – a type of ketone that is familiar, because it is used to strip remove polish.)

Not all low-carb regimens put dieters into ketosis, since you have to get below a certain carbohydrate level (which varies somewhat from one person to the next) for that to happen. The carb level assigned by The Zone, for instance, would be unlikely to put anyone into ketosis. And even diets such as the Atkins plan, which include an induction phase of severe carbohydrate restriction that leads to ketosis, don't require dieters to stay there forever. When dieters begin adding carbs back in the later phases of the diet, most stop being ketotic.

However, there is little doubt that entering a state of ketosis represents a profound metabolic change for most people. "I talk about it as if it were a drug because I think it has a druglike effect on the body," says Eric Westman, M.D., a Duke University researcher who conducted two recent studies on low-carb diets. The first looked at a group of people on low-carb diets; the second compared people on the

Atkins diet to those on conventional diets over a six-month period. In the latter case, those on the low-carb diet on average lost more weight and had more improvements in their blood lipid levels than those on the conventional diet. However, they also reported many more side effects.

Among these side effects noted by researchers were dehydration, diarrhea, fatigue, muscle cramps, and orthostatic hypotension (which means that your blood pressure drops rapidly when you stand up, making you dizzy). There have also been reports of electrolyte imbalances, cardiac arrhythmias, and dizziness.

Westman believes many of the side effects may be due not to the ketosis itself but to dehydration, something that's common in the early phases of low-carb diets. That's because for every gram of glycogen your body tucks away—glycogen being the stored form of glucose—it also stores three grams of water.

As your body rips through its glycogen stores, however, all the water that has been tied up in the storage process is released. "That's why people on low-carb diets often have a pretty substantial weight loss just in the first few days," says Lupton. (Some low-carb dieters report losing as much as ten pounds in the first week or two—although they also tend to spend a lot of time in the bathroom urinating because of this large release of water.)

Atkins called ketosis "one of life's charmed gifts . . . It's as delightful as sex and sunshine, and it has fewer drawbacks than either of them," he wrote in the 1992 edition of his book.

But one of the concerns many experts have about ketosis is that no one has studied the effects of remaining in that state for a prolonged period of time. "There's nothing that says it is [bad for you]; on the other hand, it's so abnormal that it's hard to believe it's good," says Marion Nestle, Ph.D., a professor of nutrition sciences at New York University. "I mean, it's what happens when people are starving to death."

And while none of the low-carb diets necessarily prescribe ketosis for the long term, not everyone follows the diets as they're intended. "That's what makes these things so difficult to study," says Diane Stadler, Ph.D., of Oregon Health & Science University. "When you're looking at a free-living population of people, they don't necessarily do what you tell them—they do what they want."

Saturated Fats vs. Unsaturated Fats

There are many different types of fats, but, generally speaking, they fall into four broad categories.

- *Saturated fats* come mostly from animal products. The word "saturated" refers to the fact that if you could look at its molecular structure under a microscope, you would see that it was "saturated" with hydrogen molecules. At room temperature, saturated fats are solid. (Think of a stick of butter, the fat marbled through a prime piece of beef, or the fat from bacon hardening on a cool frying pan.) A high intake of saturated fats has been linked to heart disease and possibly some cancers, so most experts advise limiting their intake. Although a low-carb diet does not have to be high in saturated fat, many are, because dieters replace carbs with animal protein and cheese. This is one of the reasons that many experts worry about the long-term effects of low-carb diets.

- *Monounsaturated fats* come largely from plant sources. Their molecular structures contain fewer hydrogen molecules than saturated fats. Monounsaturated fats are good for you, but polyunsaturated fats (see below) are better. Monounsaturated fats are liquid at room temperature, but if you put them in the refrigerator, they start to thicken. Examples of monounsaturated fats include olive oil, canola oil, and the oils contained in nuts.

- *Polyunsaturated fats* come from plant sources, just like monounsaturated fats. But polyunsaturated fats are liquid both at room temperature and when you chill them. Corn oil is polyunsaturated; so is soybean oil and the fats found in fish, such as salmon.

- *Trans-fats* are essentially man-made fats. They involve forcing hydrogen gas through a fat in the presence of a metal, usually nickel, to alter its chemical structure. This makes them solid at room temperature— something that makes them easier to ship and store. Trans-fats have been strongly linked to heart disease. By January 2006, foods containing trans-fats must include that information on their nutrition labels.

3.

Weighty Issues: Do You Really Lose More on a Low-Carb Diet?

Many studies have reported that people on low-carb diets lose more weight than those on conventional diets, at least in the short term. As a result, many of us have come to view them as magic bullets that will solve our weight problems once and for all.

There are a couple of dangers in that way of thinking, however. One is that while low-carb diets seem to take weight off easily for many people, there's still a lot of effort involved in keeping it off. Secondly, you have to remember that when study results are reported, they're usually in the form of averages. They may give a good picture of what happened to the group as a whole, but they don't do much to predict the results of an individual dieter. In other words: While some people lose a lot of weight on conventional diets, others do not.

This was illustrated by one of the first studies to come out on the subject, published in 2002 by researchers at Duke University. Of the forty-one participants, thirty-nine lost weight, and two did not. Of those who did lose, the amount varied widely, from about eight pounds to more than forty, with the average being about seventeen pounds.

Bill and Jaynelle Tenor provide another case in point. When this New Jersey couple went on the Atkins diet several years ago, Jaynelle, an adult-ed teacher in her mid-forties, was hoping to lose twenty pounds. Bill, an electronics technician who is a few years younger, wanted to shed about thirty.

Within the first couple of weeks of cutting carbs, Jaynelle took off five or six pounds and continued to lose slowly but steadily after that. "I wouldn't say the pounds melted away, but I was losing fast enough to keep me motivated," she said. After six months, she was within five pounds of her goal weight, and although she never did manage to get rid of those last few pounds, she says it was probably her own fault— she wasn't all that strict about following the diet.

Bill was a different story. Although both he and Jaynelle agree that he was far more disciplined than she was about watching his carbs, his experience wasn't nearly as good as hers. He lost only ten of the thirty pounds he was trying to take off, and it took him the full six months to do that. "A lot of people say you lose a lot of weight really fast," he says. "That never happened for me."

No one fully understands the reasons for such differences, although it could have to do with a variety of things: metabolic differences among individual dieters, how many calories they're taking in, how much exercise they're getting.

The Eades point this out in the introduction to *Protein Power*: "[W]e are all as different biochemically as we are in appearance. Every doctor has encountered patients in whom medicines seem to work in an opposite fashion to that intended, patients who are kept awake by sleeping pills and pass out on stimulants. These and similar experiences keep practiced physicians from ever making blanket this-will-ever-work-in-all-circumstances statements."

However, that doesn't mean that low-carb diets don't work. They do—although no one knows exactly why.

Atkins always insisted that a "metabolic" advantage was created by cutting carbohydrates.

"Burning fat takes more energy, so you expend more calories when you follow a controlled carbohydrate nutritional approach," he wrote.

But not everyone agrees that any such advantage exists. Some researchers theorize that the real reason low-carb dieters seem to have more initial success is that ketones take the edge off people's hunger. Others think that fat and protein are more satiating than carbs, so dieters stop eating sooner. Low-carb dieters may have another built-in psychological advantage as well, because they typically lose a lot of water weight early on, which tends to motivate them to keep going.

And even though their weight loss slows down when it comes time to start taking off actual fat, they're already so far ahead of the curve by then that it's easy to stay there, as long as they don't take in so many carbs that they begin packing on glycogen and water once again.

As evidence that water weight makes up the bulk of the extra pounds dieters lose on low-carb plans, some experts point to a study done in the mid-1970s by researchers at Columbia University. It differed from most of the studies that have been done on low-carb diets in that it was what is known as a "metabolic-ward" study. That means that instead of simply counseling subjects about what to eat and sending them home to follow through—as is the case in most diet studies—researchers hospitalized the half-dozen male participants for the entire fifty days of the study. That gave them the ability to control everything the subjects ate (in this case, a liquid diet), and to monitor its impact on their bodies by continuously testing their blood, urine, and feces. The subjects were also weighed at exactly the same time each day.

During the course of the Columbia study, each man was placed on three different liquid diets. The first was low-carb, the second was a regular "mixed" diet that included a normal proportion of carbs to fat and protein, and the third was the equivalent of a fast. Researchers found that on average, subjects actually burned a tiny (although probably statistically insignificant) bit *more* fat on the "mixed" diet than they did on the low-carb diet—166 grams versus 163 grams per day. But the overall weight loss on the low-carb diet was greater because the subjects lost so much more water.

The results are similar to those of a few other early metabolic-ward studies done on low-carb diets. However, the results differed markedly from those of a 1965 study often quoted by Atkins as proof that low-carb diets burn more fat. In that study—also done on a metabolic ward—researchers at the Oakland Naval Hospital found that men who were placed on low-carb diet of 1,000 calories a day lost a little more than a pound per day, and that nearly 98 percent of that weight loss was fat. The Columbia researchers, on the other hand, found that only 35 percent of the weight their patients lost was fat—an amount similar to that lost on all the other studies, except the one by the Oakland team. That caused some scientists to question the results of the Oakland study. They said they weren't convinced the subjects could have burned that much fat without vigorous exercise—something that would be difficult for do while confined to a hospital ward.

However, William Yancy, M.D., of Duke University, says that if the metabolic-ward studies had lasted longer, they might have had different results, because once people get past the first couple of weeks, the composition of their weight loss seems to change from largely water to largely fat. "In our study, [participants] lost a total of twenty-six pounds over six months, but seventy-five percent of that was fat," says Yancy. "So while water loss is definitely a factor at first, it doesn't seem to bear true in the longer-duration studies."

He and coresearcher Eric Westman, M.D., believe that one of the reasons the low-carb group in their studies lost more weight is that ketones themselves have an appetite-suppressing effect. "People told me they just weren't hungry," Westman says. As a result, they may have been eating less on the diet.

An experiment set up by the British Broadcasting Corporation for a science documentary seems to bear out Westman and Yancy's hypothesis. For the program, 240 people were assigned to one of four diets: a conventional low-fat, low-calorie diet; Weight Watchers; Slim-Fast; or the Atkins Plan. They were also asked to keep detailed diaries of what they ate, and were followed (and filmed) for a year. At first, the dieters on the Atkins plan lost a lot more weight than the others, but by the end of the year, everyone else had caught up. Producers hired scientists to analyze the data, and they reported that—if the food diaries were to be believed—the Atkins dieters consistently consumed fewer calories than the others.

Some of the most convincing evidence that a calorie is just a calorie, however, comes from a 2001 study done jointly by Diane Stadler and Njeri Karanja, Ph.D., a nutrition researcher at the Kaiser Permanente Health Research Center in Portland.

Their team wanted to see what would happen if two groups of dieters were to consume exactly the same amount of calories but differing amounts of fat and carbohydrates. Backed by funding from the National Institutes of Health, they started out by putting twenty-five people who were obese but otherwise healthy on the induction phase of the Atkins diet.

In most of the low-carb studies done to date, researchers have simply talked to subjects about the sorts of foods allowed on the diet and sent them home to follow through. Participants shop for their own food and prepare their own meals, then fill out detailed forms about what they've eaten—something that's notoriously inaccurate, since people don't always remember (or confess) everything they consume. As a result, their caloric intake tends to be significantly underreported.

The Oregon study, however, was different. It was what was known as a "metabolic feeding study"— meaning that instead of sending participants home to fend for themselves, the researchers actually supplied all of their food for the first six weeks. Such studies aren't done often because they are phenomenally expensive and time-consuming, but they do have an advantage over other types of studies in that researchers can monitor exactly how much and what type of food participants eat, and also make sure everyone is eating the same thing. "It's a very tightly controlled study," Stadler explains.

The first step was to figure out exactly how many calories each participant required on a daily basis in order to maintain his or her weight, a calculation made on the basis of body mass index (BMI), age, sex, and activity level. Each day, participants were given Atkins-style meals and snacks which contained 20 percent more calories than they were estimated to need, but only twenty grams of carbohydrates. They were allowed to eat as much or as little of the food as they wanted, but had to bring the rest back to the medical center the next day so researchers could reweigh it, thereby calculating the precise number of calories each person had consumed.

On average, the researchers found, Atkins dieters ate only 70 percent of the calories needed each day to maintain their weight. "If they'd eaten everything we gave them, they almost certainly would have gained weight," said Stadler. "So the fact that they were restricting their caloric intake by themselves by thirty percent – that's really impressive."

Armed with that data, the researchers then moved into the second phase of the study. That meant feeding twenty-five addtional healthy but obese subjects the precise number of calories the Atkins group had been eating—in other words, about 70 percent of what they were calculated to need on a daily basis.

But the new group of dieters—who were carefully matched to the Atkins group in terms of BMI, sex, lipid profile, and other parameters—received those calories in the form of a diet known as DASH—short for Dietary Approaches to Solving Hypertension. As its name indicates, this diet was designed primarily to help people lower their blood pressure, not to lose weight, although people who go on it do tend to lose a little weight. It contains less sodium than most diets, along with plenty of fruits, vegetables, and whole grains, and gets 55 percent of its calories from carbs, 18 percent from protein, and 27 percent from fat, which qualifies it as a low-fat diet, but not an extreme one. "We chose it because it's kind of a gold standard for a conventional healthy diet," Stadler explains.

Like the Atkins group, the DASH dieters were supplied with all of their food for the first six weeks of the study. But unlike the Atkins group, who were told to eat only as much as they wanted to, the DASH dieters were told that they had to eat everything they were given each day.

Both they and the Atkins group reported to the clinic daily for a weigh-in and a check of their blood pressure; they also had to provide a urine sample. At least weekly, researchers also checked their blood lipids, and they periodically tested the dieter's bone density and kidney function as well. The participants received food for only six weeks, but researchers followed them for an additional twelve to see how they'd do on their own. And after a year, the team checked back in as well.

The data they collected showed that both groups lost the same amount of weight during the first six weeks of the study, and lost it at the same rate— about two pounds a week. Both were also able to maintain that weight loss through the eighteen-week mark. And both lost mostly fat, as opposed to lean body mass.

Although Atkins officials claimed a victory in that study, noting in a press kit that Atkins dieters lost an average of 14.3 pounds while the DASH group lost 11.4 pounds, researchers said the difference was not statistically significant. Their conclusion? "If caloric intake is the same, weight loss is the same—that was our bottom line," Stadler says.

The other bottom line—not only with the Oregon study but with all those studies that have followed low-carb dieters for at least a year—is that over the long haul, the low-carb dieters don't seem to do any better than conventional dieters. In other words, for a diet to work, you have to be able to stick to it. And while that's an individual factor to some degree, when scientists have followed large groups of people who've kept the weight off, they've noted that they all had certain things in common. Those include: regular exercise; "self-monitoring" (meaning that they keep tabs on their weight); eating a low-fat, low-calorie diet; and not skipping breakfast. In fact, statistics from the National Weight Control Registry, a database of people eighteen years of age and older who have lost at least thirty pounds on a low-carb diet and kept it off for a year, found that 1 percent of those registered are on low-carb diets. (That, of course, may be because people on low-carb diets simply haven't bothered to put their names on the registry; another registry specifically for low-carb dieters was recently set up at Albert Einstein Medical Center in New York.)

What registry data suggest is that most people on

the registry have certain things in common: They exercise regularly and eat a low-fat diet, getting an average of about 23 percent of their calories from fat. They also tend to take smaller portions of whatever they eat, consume fewer snacks, and don't indulge in butter, cheese, fried foods, or desserts more than once a week, the registry has found.

As for the Tenors, the New Jersey couple that had differing experiences on the Atkins plan, both ended up going off it after six months, because they were traveling almost every weekend and, at that time, there weren't many low-carb options available in restaurants, which made it hard for them to feed themselves and stay low-carb on the road.

It wasn't easy preparing the right low-carb food at home, either. "I wish I had time to get up in the morning and make a cheese omelet before I went to work, but it's just not in my schedule," says Jaynelle, a mother of three who also works full-time and raises and shows horses. Still, she says, some of the effects of her low-carb experience have lingered. "Before, we ate quite a bit of rice and potatoes, and we haven't really gotten back into that," she says. "I don't buy potatoes anymore, unless I'm making something special with them; I don't eat that much pasta anymore. So I think it's still affecting our diet in some ways."

Overall, she liked the diet a lot, she says, and she's thinking about going on it again, trying to lose the dozen or so pounds that have crept back on since her Atkins days.

But Bill says that this time he won't be joining her. "It's just not the right diet for me," he says.

4.

The Heart of the Matter

In the autumn of 2003, a Florida businessman named Jody Gorran was told by his cardiologist that one of his coronary arteries was 99 percent clogged and would require angioplasty to open it.

In a country where heart disease affects nearly one out of every two people, it was a run-of-the-mill diagnosis—the sort given to thousands of people every month, and certainly not anything you'd expect to make the evening news. But Gorran's case did make national news, because of what happened next: He filed a lawsuit against Atkins Nutritionals, the company founded by the late cardiologist Robert Atkins, alleging that the diet it promoted gave him heart disease.

While there have been heated discussions as to the merits of Gorran's case, it did bring out a point that seems to have gotten lost in our rush toward the low-carb aisle at the grocery store: Virtually every study done on low-carb diets has shown that while many people do seem to have an improvement in cholesterol and triglycerides after going on a low-carb diet, between a quarter and a third of dieters not only don't get better, they get worse.

Although that's sometimes hard to discern, based on the way the studies are reported in the popular press, it was clearly illustrated by a study published in 2002 by researchers at Duke University. Of the forty-one people in the study, twelve had an increase in their LDL cholesterol, generally considered "bad" cholesterol because of its tendency to stick to arterial walls. (Two more had increases and were concerned enough by them that they quit the study.) Researchers noted that one subject had an LDL that zoomed from 123 to 225 while on the low-carb diet but went back down to 176 after the participant began taking cholesterol-lowering nutritional supplements. And in another 2003 report comparing various blood markers in fourteen people with type 2 diabetes, three had increases in their total cholesterol levels.

"If you have eighteen people in a room and a third of them have a really bad reaction to something and two thirds don't, that's not what I'd call a good result," says Neal Barnard, M.D., president and founder of Physicians Committee for Responsible Medicine, a group that actively promotes a vegetarian diet and has gone head-to-head with Atkins on numerous occasions. "If a drug caused a cholesterol increase like this, it would be pulled off the market."

But part of the problem with discussing the impact of heart disease on low-carb diets stems from the fact that—as is the case with so many other aspects of the diet debate—the science isn't clear on either side.

Pro-carb advocates point out that decades of studies have shown a link between saturated fat and heart disease, and that possibility isn't written off by all low-carb diet doctors. Arthur Agatston, M.D., writes that the reason the South Beach Diet recommends only unsaturated fats is because studies have shown that after eating even one meal that's high in saturated fat, the lining of arteries becomes temporarily "predisposed to constriction and clotting."

"Imagine," he writes, "under the right (or rather, wrong) circumstances, eating a meal that's high in saturated fat can trigger a heart attack!"

But other low-carb advocates maintain that problems arise only if carbs are present along with the saturated fat, and cite a number of studies that suggest this—including some of the same studies cited by pro-carbers as "proof" that low-carb diets are dangerous to heart health—the difference being that they concentrate on the patients who had improvements in their serum lipid levels, while critics concentrate on those who didn't.

The debate blew up while Atkins was still alive, when a Nebraska cardiologist named Richard Fleming published a study of twenty-six patients with heart disease whom he planned to track for a year. The patients were advised to eat diets that were extremely low in fat, but not all of them complied; ten actually went on low-carb diets of one form or another because they believed they would "improve" their health, Fleming wrote in a published report of the study, which appeared in the October 2000 issue of the *International Journal of Angiology*. The results of a series of tests found that heart disease regressed in the patients on the low-fat diet and progressed in the patients on the low-carb diets.

Atkins appeared on the Today show to complain about it. "This was not a study of the low-carbohydrate diet," he said. "This was [a study of] a group of people who cheated . . . If you eat protein and carbohydrates, you don't do well. But if you cut out carbohydrates, you do dramatically better."

Although everyone on both sides of the debate agrees that LDL does go up in some people on low-carb diets, they don't agree on the significance of an increase of LDL in some people on the diet. Some say any increase in cholesterol should be taken seriously. Others say we should be comparing the ratio of HDL to triglycerides, not to LDL, if we want a more accurate picture of heart-disease risk—although, again, that ratio doesn't improve in all people on low-carb diets. (In the 2003 report, it improved in eleven patients, stayed the same in one, and got a little worse in two.)

And still others tend to focus on VLDL—short for "very low density lipoprotein," a subtype of LDL molecule that is big and fluffy and therefore less likely to cause problems than smaller, denser, "regular" LDL molecules. They point out that some studies have found that many—but again not all—people on low-carb diets tend to have a better ratio of VLDL to regular LDL.

"This whole lipid issue is really complex," says *Protein Power*'s Michael Eades, who, like a growing number of other experts, isn't even convinced that blood lipids are a very good predictor of heart disease. "If it were, half the people who have heart attacks wouldn't have normal cholesterol," says Eades. He thinks heart disease may have more to do with inflammation than cholesterol, a view shared by a growing number of researchers, and he points out that markers for inflammation also tend to improve for many patients when they go on low-carb diets—although, once again, that varies from one person the next.

But Diane Stadler, Ph.D., of Oregon Health & Sciences University, says she doesn't think that we're at a point where we can afford to ignore changes in cholesterol and triglycerides. In the study she worked on—like virtually all of the others—a "not insignificant" number of participants had lipid levels that got much worse, and the change was noticeable within two weeks of going on the diet, Stadler says.

"This is something that needs to be taken seriously," she added. "Some people are going to respond okay, and that's great. But others aren't, and you need to identify those people and intervene early, either by taking them off the diet or putting them on appropriate medications." It will also be important to keep checking in with them as they continue on low-carb diets, since the longest time to date that low-carb dieters have been studied has been a year, she said.

Although most people still evidenced improvements in their blood lipid levels at that time, "We just don't have enough data to say what happens beyond that," says Samuel Klein, M.D., the Danforth Professor of Medicine and Nutritional Sciences at Washington University in St. Louis, and an internationally known researcher on obesity and weight loss.

Klein is now working on a government-funded study that will follow dieters for five years. Asked whether there was any reason to think that lipid levels that have been stable for a year might change after that, Klein said it is "certainly possible," although it is more likely to be due to a compliance issue than a physiological one. "For example, if [dieters] started eating more carbohydrates and calories and maintained a high fat intake, things could get worse. But we don't have data yet. We really do need long-term, more comprehensive studies to fully evaluate the effectiveness of this approach," he said.

In the 1992 and 1998 editions of his book, Atkins himself noted the fact that not everyone's risk profile for heart disease seemed to respond the same way to a low-carb diet. "I will admit that there are individuals who are fat-sensitive and will develop a less favorable cholesterol level on a high-fat diet than on a low-fat diet," he wrote in a section titled Good Protection for Your Heart, which has been omitted from the 2002 edition of the book. "Intensive study of medical reports strongly suggests that fewer than one person in three falls into this category."

He suggested that the one in three who does experience elevated cholesterol readings try a lower-fat version of the diet, choosing leaner cuts of meat, such as turkey roll and skinless chicken breast, and have their lipids rechecked. "However, if you're not happy on the low-fat version of the diet or get hungry or don't feel as well on it, then don't bother with it; go back to the regular Atkins diet that you enjoyed more," he added. He also recommended that such persons take nutritional supplements, including vitamin C, chromium picolinate, and pantethine, which he said usually lower blood lipids to levels "satisfactory enough" to make cholesterol-lowering medications unnecessary.

"Nowhere," says Gorran, "does he say to get off the diet."

Jody Gorran, the 53-year-old businessman whose
company manufactures solar heaters for swimming
pools, says he went on the Atkins diet in May 2001,
hoping to take off about ten pounds and prevent
middle-age spread. Although he knew that most
medical experts believe a high intake of saturated fat
could lead to atherosclerosis and heart disease, he
was satisfied with the way Atkins addressed the
issue. "Of the many misconceptions that surround
the Atkins Nutritional Approach, perhaps the most
widespread is the assumption that eating foods high
in fat is a health risk," the company's website says.
"Not so—in the absence of refined carbohydrates."

It then goes on to cite numerous studies that
support this, including one done by researchers at
Ball State University, in which a dozen men who
followed the Atkins plan for two months managed to
lower their cholesterol by an average of 55 percent.
Gorran was impressed with the body of evidence
Atkins presented. "The theory made sense to me,"
Gorran says. "I thought he knew something that
nobody else knew."

So in May 2001, Gorran slashed carbohydrates
from his diet and was thrilled with the results.
Although he was still able to eat his favorite foods,
such as steak and cheesecake (made according to an

Atkins recipe, without a crust and with artificial sweetener), he lost weight quickly, exactly as Atkins's book had promised.

"I told everyone who would listen how great it was," Gorran recalls. True, his cholesterol went up sharply—from 146 to 230—within six months of starting the plan. But the Atkins book had given him the impression that this wasn't something he had to be concerned about, he said, so he didn't—especially since a few months before going on the diet, he'd had a complete physical, including a CT scan of his coronary arteries. The scan had shown his arteries to be perfectly clear—meaning that his chances of developing heart disease in the next few years were almost zilch. "So I wasn't really worried," Gorran says. Nor did he worry about the implications for his own health when his sister—who had a cholesterol reading of 250, even though she was following a low-fat diet—had a heart attack. "I thought I was protected," Gorran explains. "I was on the low-carb diet."

Then, in October 2003, when he'd been on the diet about a year and a half, he and his wife traveled to New York City for a long weekend visit with their son, who lived there. Gorran's wife wanted to go shopping—not Gorran's favorite activity—so he set out on foot along Manhattan's Fifth Avenue for a day of museum hopping.

It was cool and sunny— a perfect day for walking. But Gorran had gone only about a quarter mile when he noticed a strange, heavy sensation in his chest—almost as if someone were grinding a fist into it. Startled, he stood still and the feeling disappeared. But it came back as soon as he started walking again, so he hailed a taxi to take him the rest of the way to the museum. "It went away the minute I got in the cab," he recalled.

Later that night, as Gorran and his wife hurried through a theater lobby, the weird feeling came back. And on his way home from a business trip a week or two later, as he hustled through an airport terminal carrying nothing heavier than an overnight bag, it got so bad that he had to stop. "It was [a feeling of] real pressure," he recalled. "Like something was pushing on my heart."

Really worried now, Gorran called his doctor, who said it sounded suspiciously like angina and referred him to a cardiologist. A series of tests, including another CT scan, revealed the blockage in one of his main arteries, as well as smaller blockages in others. He was lucky, the cardiologist told him— most people don't discover they have such a problem until they keel over from a heart attack.

Gorran was stunned. "I went from no blockage to ninety-nine-point-five percent blockage in a major artery in two and a half years," he says. "I came really close to dying—and all because of this damn diet. I was misled and betrayed."

Gorran underwent an angioplasty to clear the blockage, and now has a permanent stent in his artery to keep it open. On his doctor's orders, he also began eating a low-fat diet with lots of lean meats, fruits, vegetables, and whole grains. Within a few weeks, his cholesterol dropped from the 209 it had tested at right before the angioplasty to 146—exactly where it had been before he'd gone on the low-carb plan. "That proved to me that the whole thing was related to diet," Gorran says. "I was eating things I'd never eaten before."

In his lawsuit, filed last spring, Gorran asks for only $15,000—money he says he'll donate to charity if he wins. The point, he says, isn't to get rich—it's to bring attention to the fact that the diet isn't necessarily as safe for everyone as the headlines make it seem. "You cannot ignore a third of the people," he insists. "It's unethical."

Not surprisingly, perhaps, Atkins representatives fired right back, saying Gorran was the one who was questionable. "If he has a true and valid concern, his case should be reviewed by nutritional experts," says Stuart L. Trager, M.D., the company's medical director. "And this should not be done by inflammatory, anecdotal reporting . . . but through case reports, medical literature—the kind of peer-reviewed, nonbiased, evidence-based medicine that affects change."

Trager, who calls the lawsuit "frivolous" and "a distraction," says he particularly objects to the fact that Gorran's suit is being paid for by PCRM, which is the same group that released the coroner's report on Atkins to the media.

"They are a horrible group," he says.

Barnard returns the compliment. "They [Atkins's company] like to cast aspersions on us, but I am quite happy to defend who I am and what our organization is to anything they might wish to say," he says. "Yes, it's true that we advocate exactly the opposite diet from them. But what we are doing is honest and correct. Their only goal is to sell things."

He pauses, then adds wryly: "I'd love to take them in, give them some oatmeal and a bean burrito. In a month I'd have them singing 'Kumbaya.' "

In its response to Gorran's lawsuit, attorneys for Atkins Nutritionals have filed a motion for dismissal. In a statement, the company says Gorran "clearly ignored key sentences next to those he quotes as evidence of wrongdoing."

The statement points out that in the same section of the book quoted in Gorran's lawsuit, Atkins also told dieters that "[t]o perfect your lipid levels you have to be willing to have the blood tests analyzed frequently; otherwise, you are as guilty as those consensus-formers, always assuming everybody's metabolic response is the same. The strategy is to systematically test our various hypotheses and then look at blood test results to see if they are operative for you."

The statement also says Atkins advised dieters whose lipids went down on the lower-fat version of the diet to switch back to the high-fat version, then do another blood test to see if the lipid level goes back up again. "If it bounced back up from the previous one, then you are fat-sensitive and should follow the fat-restricted variation of the diet," Atkins wrote.

Not only did Gorran not pay attention to that part of the book, Trager says, but by choosing to address his concerns through a highly publicized lawsuit instead of accepted scientific channels, he "is hurting the millions of people who can be helped by this [low-carb] approach."

But Gorran is unperturbed by such charges. He says that he did read the book carefully, and that if he misunderstood what Atkins was saying—which he doesn't think he did—it's likely that other people did, too.

Besides, he says, if the diet helps some people, that's fine; he doesn't think it should be banned. He just wants people to know that not everyone responds to it the same way, and would like to see a warning label saying as much on both the book and related products. "If Atkins wants to settle the suit for something like that, I'd consider it," he says.

Clinton and South Beach

The issue of low-carb diets and heart health, which seemed to be fading in the wake of some of the new studies, was back in the headlines last summer, thanks to former President Bill Clinton. The former chief executive, who had a well-known junk-food habit, had gone on the wildly popular South Beach Det earlier in the year and had lost a noticeable amount of weight, reportedly even going off his cholesterol-lowering medication.

But over Labor Day weekend of 2004, he began experiencing shortness of breath. Tests revealed major blockages in his coronary arteries, and he was immediately hospitalized for quadruple bypass surgery.

The news set off immediate speculation in some pro-carb quarters that Clinton's recent foray into low-carb dieting might have played a role. John A. McDougall, M.D., author of *The McDougall Program for Maximum Weight Loss* and several other books promoting a high-carb, low-fat diet, addressed this in an open letter he wrote to the president: "Your most recent attempt at weight loss, the South Beach Diet, contributed to your present troubles. Steak, chicken, eggs, and Canadian bacon consumed without limitation are bad for your arteries, Bill."

The publicist for South Beach creator Arthur Agatston, M.D., did not respond to a request for an interview. But when Agatston, a cardiologist, was asked by a CNN interviewer at the time of Clinton's surgery whether it was possible that the former president's problem was connected to the South Beach Diet, Agatston denied it firmly. "Not at all," he said. "We're low in processed carbohydrates, the bad carbs. . . . We're very high in vegetables and whole fruits, whole grains that have been shown to diminish heart disease." Rather, he said—and most experts agreed with him—Clinton's problem "grew up over a lifetime. . . . What he needed was early diagnosis with a heart scan, which could have picked up the disease developing five, ten years ago. And then he could have been on the proper medication, as well as diet and exercise."

The Death of Rachel Huskey

In the summer of 2000, Rachel Huskey, a sixteen-year-old high-school honor student from Sturgeon, Missouri, saw an infomercial on the Atkins diet and excitedly ordered the videotapes. Pretty but a little on the chubby side, she was, as her father, Paul, puts it, "at that age where she wanted to be attractive to boys," and with its promise of quick results and appealing list of permissible foods, the high-protein, low-carb eating plan seemed to be the answer.

It didn't take Rachel long to lose fifteen pounds on the diet, Paul Huskey says, and while she went off the diet a couple months later when the family went away on vacation, she went back on it again just before school started in August.

Eight days later, the phone rang. It was Rachel's school, telling Huskey and his wife, Lisa, that they needed to get there right away. "They wouldn't tell us what was wrong," Huskey recalls.

The couple rushed to the school, where they

learned that Rachel had collapsed during history class. When EMTs arrived, they discovered that her heart was beating in an erratic pattern typically seen in adults who've suffered heart attacks. Rachel was airlifted to the hospital but was pronounced dead later that day.

In a report on the case published in a medical journal, Rachel's doctor, D. Paul Robinson, M.D., an assistant professor of child health at the University of Missouri-Columbia, said the cause of death was an arrhythmia triggered by dangerously low levels of sodium, calcium, and potassium in her blood.

While there was no way to prove that the problem was due to the diet she was following, Robinson said, "Our findings are consistent with what we understand is the body's potential response to [the diet]."

Atkins's medical director Stuart L. Trager, M.D., calls Rachel's death "tragic," but says he questions whether it really was diet-related. "None of these studies in which people have been followed, not in one of them has there ever been a metabolic abnormality like that," he says, adding that dieters should be checking in with their doctors anyway.

That makes Huskey angry. "On the tapes it said if you have health problems consult your physician.

If you don't have health problems, you're fine. Rachel didn't have anything wrong with her—just tree allergies, that's all. She was never sick." He pauses, "There's a big loss in our life, a big hole that will never be filled," he says. "We'll never see Rachel go to college, get married, see the grandchildren that would have been from her. All that's over just because of a simple diet. You know, one thing I'd really like to tell everybody out there is, losing a few pounds is not worth risking your life for on any diet. Know what the risks are before you start."

5.

The Long–Term Effects

ost of the studies done to date on low-carb diets have focused on how they impact participants' weight and heart-disease risk. But what we eat affects a lot more than that. It influences virtually every aspect of our health, in ways that may not be apparent for years to come. No wonder, then, that when it comes to a discussion of the long-term impact of low-carb diets, the fighting really begins.

While even critics concede that cutting carbs hasn't been shown to be harmful to most people in the short term, they point out that there's a big difference between eating something for a little while and eating it for the rest of your life.

"You could eat the bark off a pine tree for six months and be okay," says Suzanne Havala-Hobbs, a clinical assistant professor in the Department of Health Policy and Administration at the University of North Carolina's School of Public Health. "It's what you do long-term that is of relevance."

The list of problems that she and other critics fear might be caused by cutting carbs reads like a public-health nightmare: cancer, kidney stones, kidney disease, osteoporosis, gout, and even vision problems. But some of those are chronic diseases that take decades to develop and can't be accurately assessed in the sort of short-term studies that have been done so far on low-carb diets. "Are we going to see an increase in colon cancer twenty years down the line because people aren't getting enough fiber?" asks Barbara Moore, Ph.D., president of Shape Up America!, a nonprofit group dedicated to helping Americans achieve permanent weight loss. "Are we going to see more kidney disease or osteoporosis? I don't think anybody really knows the answer yet. We've essentially embarked on a huge societal experiment with this diet, and who knows what price we're going to pay."

But fans pooh-pooh such projections as scare tactics, and claim that even if such risks existed— something they dispute—they'd be more than offset by the benefits of losing weight. "The real enemy here is obesity and overweight," says Collette Heimowitz, director of education and research for Atkins Nutritionals, pointing out that extra weight itself has been linked to many of the same health problems that critics say could be caused by low-carb diets. "People need viable options to achieve losing their excess weight, and that's all this is," she says. "It's a tool."

In the eyes of critics, the problem lies with both what low-carb diets contain (saturated fat) and what they don't (sufficient quantities of fruits and vegetables, which contain both fiber and micronutrients). The former has been strongly linked to some cancers; the latter seem to protect against them. But no one has direct data to prove this. Rather, each side's claims are based on data extrapolated from nutritional studies that were being done to look at things other than low-carb diets—and data that low-carb proponents insist may not be valid when carbs are extracted from the equation.

The problem is that doing the right studies will take time and money—if they can be done at all. It's relatively easy to measure something like heart-disease risk using a randomized, controlled study—a type of study that involves putting two groups of people on two different regimen, and comparing how each responds—because there's something you can measure in the short term: Either your cholesterol and triglycerides go up or they don't. But trying to do such a study to determine cancer would be bankruptingly expensive (if it could be done at all), because the study would have to go on for so long and would require so many participants to be accurate.

That means that the only way to study such problems is through an epidemiological study. In this type of study, also known as a longitudinal study, large groups of people are followed loosely over long periods of time. But there are built-in problems with such studies, because they rely a great deal on participants' memory of particular events—what they've eaten over the previous year, for instance, or how many colds they've had. For instance, many doctors prescribed hormone-replacement therapy to menopausal women because epidemiological studies indicated that it helped prevent heart disease. But when a randomized, controlled study was done, it found that HRT might actually cause heart disease.

"One of the underlying problems in this whole discussion is that there's no perfect study," says

Harvard's Walter Willett, M.D. "If we're just looking at weight alone, it's no problem, because you can measure that directly by studying a relatively small group of people for a year or two. You don't need tens of thousands of people over decades, like you do with cancer."

With that in mind, it is important to examine the concerns people have about the long-term impact of low-carb diets, and why they have them.

Osteoporosis

Also known as "brittle bone disease," osteoporosis is a chronic condition characterized by bones that are fragile and break easily. The condition can be both painful and debilitating, especially when it occurs in the hip or spine. One out of two women and one out of eight men over age fifty have osteoporosis, and many experts believe that the longer you're on a low-carb diet, the greater your chances of getting it. Do they have the long-term studies proving this will happen? Well, no. But here's why they're still concerned.

All low-carbohydrate diets are somewhat higher in protein than the average diet. That's because when you cut carbs from your diet, you have to replace them with something, and one of your only two choices is protein. (The other is fat.) When you eat protein, your stomach and intestines break it down into amino acids, which your body will use to rebuild and repair itself. But when you get more protein than your body can use, you end up with a lot more amino acids than usual in your blood, which makes your blood more acidic than your body would like it to be. To prevent that from occurring and throwing all sorts of things off-kilter, your body neutralizes it using minerals, particularly calcium. Where does it get the calcium? Well, at least some of it comes from your bones.

In one long-term study that looked at a large group of women over a period of more than a decade, for instance, Harvard researchers found that those who ate more than ninety-five grams of protein a day—that's the equivalent of about two hamburgers – were 20 percent more likely to have suffered a wrist fracture than those who ate an average amount of protein (defined as about sixty-five grams per day).

Protein Power author Michael Eades doesn't dismiss the concerns about osteoporosis. But he believes some of the risk depends on exactly what people are eating. A diet that is very heavy in hard cheeses, meats, and grains—all of which are acid-forming foods—will take its toll over time, he says. "You could develop osteoporosis if you eat a diet like that." But he believes eating plenty of leafy green vegetables and fruits will offset a diet like that, because the byproducts of their metabolism are alkaline, and will help to neutralize the acid, offsetting the need to draw calcium to do the same thing. "If you balance the meat and cheese by eating plenty of fruits and leafy green vegetables, I believe you'll be fine," he says.

Kidney Disease

A diet that is high in protein has the potential to affect not only the bones but also the kidneys, because they will have to work harder to deal with the biochemical changes triggered by the diet.

What does that mean? Well, probably not much if your kidneys are functioning normally. But new studies suggest that for people who have even mild kidney dysfunction—something they may not be aware of—high protein intakes can cause big problems.

Harvard researchers recently reported on 1,624 female nurses whom they've been monitoring since

1989 as part of a much larger study to determine the connection between health and lifestyle. The women regularly fill out extensive questionnaires about their diets and periodically undergo blood tests. Of the participants, 489 had mild kidney problems at the outset of the study, and researchers wanted to see whether their diet affected the progression of the problem.

Their findings? Women who didn't have kidney problems didn't seem to develop them as a result of eating a lot of protein. But women who had even mild kidney dysfunction at the outset of the study and consumed a lot of protein—particularly meat—got worse much faster than expected. (Women who got most of their protein from dairy products or vegetable sources such as soy didn't decline nearly as quickly.)

Here's the other thing that's worth knowing: As many as one in nine of us may have reduced kidney function—and most of us don't know it, according to the American Kidney Foundation. High blood pressure damages your kidneys and affects one in four adults—many of whom don't know they have it. Even age plays a role. Some studies suggest that by age forty, kidney function gradually begins to decline in most people. Do you take a lot of nonprescription painkillers, such as ibuprofen or acetaminophen? They've been shown to affect your kidneys if you take a lot of them over a long period of time, especially in combination with caffeine. "If you have even slight kidney damage—even you're not in kidney failure—you need to be careful about a high-protein diet," says Ellie Schlam, spokeswoman for the National Kidney Foundation.

Gout

Gout is one of the most painful forms of arthritis. It occurs when so much uric acid builds up in the blood that it begins to precipitate out, forming needle-sharp crystals that become lodged in the joints. Symptoms develop suddenly—often seemingly overnight—and include swelling, purplish discoloration, and pain so crippling that sufferers often cannot bear so much as the weight of a bedsheet on the affected area. The big toe is one of the most common sites of an attack of gout, but gout can also occur in the ankles, wrists, knees, or elbows. An attack can last anywhere between a few hours and a few weeks. Gout affects more men than women, and many experts believe some people have a genetic predisposition to it.

Although no studies have been done to specifically assess the incidence of gout in people who are on low-carb diets, many experts think it's likely to be higher than normal. Here's why.

Proteins, particularly those in red meat and shellfish, are high in amino acids called purines. When the body breaks them down, the by-product is uric acid. The more meat you consume, the more purines your body has to process, and the more uric acid you produce as a result. (In fact, in centuries past, gout was known as "the rich man's disease," because it affected only those wealthy enough to be able to afford large quantities of meat.)

In addition, taking off weight very quickly can also release large amounts of purines into the blood, which can in turn lead to high levels of uric acid in the blood.

In one study, researchers at Massachusetts General Hospital found that eating a diet high in meat and seafood—particularly if it was also low in dairy products, which seem to have a protective effect—clearly increased the risk of gout. However, eating vegetable protein also seemed to help protect against gout.

Kidney Stones

Kidney stones are lumps of minerals, such as calcium, that form in the kidneys. They can be as small as a grain of sand or as large as a ping-pong ball, and they're excruciatingly painful—even more so than childbirth, according to women who've experienced both. Small stones—those less than about a quarter-inch in diameter—usually pass through the urinary tract on their own, although it may take a few days for them to do so. Larger stones often become lodged in the kidney or urethra, and usually require medical intervention, such as the use of high-energy shockwaves, to break them up. Left untreated, they can lead to kidney failure.

None of the people in the low-carb diet studies done so far appear to have developed kidney stones. At Johns Hopkins Hospital, where a ketogenic diet is regularly used to control seizures in children with epilepsy, doctors report that between 5 and 8 percent of the children on the diet develop kidney stones within a year.

Many researchers believe this may happen for a number of reasons. One common type of kidney stone is formed largely of calcium, which precipitates out of the urine and crystallizes in the kidneys—and, as previously discussed, people on high-protein diets tend to have higher amounts of calcium in their urine. And a diet high in purine—a compound found in meat, fish, and protein—has long been identified as a risk factor for kidney stones because it leads to an increase in uric acid, which is a component in some kidney stones.

Mary Vernon, M.D., a Lawrence, Kansas, family practitioner and vice president of the American Society of Bariatric Physicians, has been using the Atkins Nutritional Approach with her patients for a number of years. Vernon says that she occasionally sees kidney stones in patients who are on the diet, but not at a rate any higher than she'd expect to see in the population at large. Most of the patients who do experience kidney stones also report having had them at some point before going on low-carb diets, which could mean they're more prone to them than most people, said Vernon, who is a member of the Atkins Physicians Council and coauthor of Atkins Diabetes Revolution, a book about using low-carb diets to treat type 2 diabetes.

Cancer

Studies have repeatedly suggested that eating a diet that's high in saturated fat leads to an increased risk of developing some forms of cancer, including colon cancer and even lung cancer.

For instance, in a study published in 1997, researchers at M.D. Anderson Cancer Center in Houston compared the diets of African-American and Mexican-American men. They found that those who ate the most fat and had the lowest intake of fruits and vegetables had the highest incidence of lung cancer—even if they didn't smoke. And when Harvard researchers looked at dietary records of 76,000 women as part of an ongoing study, they found that those who ate the most meat had the highest rates of colon cancer.

In addition, many low-carb diets curtail consumption of fruit and some vegetables, which are rich in micronutrients that are believed to help prevent cancer. They're also low in fiber, which is also believed to have some protective effects. Some low-carb diets recommend taking vitamin and mineral as well as fiber supplements; however, we just don't know whether the supplements have the same effect as real food.

"It could be better, it could be worse. We just don't know because all the studies that have been done have been done on the real thing, not the supplement," says Joanne Lupton of Texas A&M.

But low-carb fans point out that obesity itself may contribute to as many as 90,000 cases of cancer every year. Among them: breast cancer, lymphoma, colon cancer, endometrial cancer, cervical cancer, ovarian cancer, and even certain brain tumors.

Birth Defects

Folic acid, also known as folate, is one of the B vitamins, and it is critical to the development of the brain and spine in the fetus. Women who don't get enough of it are at higher risk of giving birth to a baby with neural-tube defects such as spina bifida. Folic acid deficiency has also been strongly linked to neuroblastoma, the most common cancer in infants and the leading cause of cancer death in children between the ages one and four. Many researchers believe it begins to develop even before birth.

Folic acid is found primarily in starchy foods such as beans, peas, wheat germ and brewer's yeast, as well as leafy, dark-green vegetables, and liver—foods that many women don't get enough of even if they're not on low-carb diets. So in an attempt to prevent such deficiency-related problems, the United States and Canada began adding it to white flour in the late 1990s. Since then, spina bifida and other neural-tube defects have plummeted by more than 30 percent; Canadian statistics also indicate that the incidence of neuroblastoma is down more than 60 percent.

But now, with a growing number of women of childbearing age avoiding folate-enriched foods, scientists worry that this trend could begin to reverse itself. Of course, a woman who is planning to become pregnant can make up for this by taking supplements. But the problem is that many pregnancies are unplanned, and beginning folic acid supplements after becoming pregnant won't help, because the folate needs to be in a woman's system when the fetus's brain and spinal cord are forming— something that occurs during the first eighteen days of pregnancy, well before many women realize they're pregnant. That means women who are counting carbs are missing a vitamin that is essential to the health of their unborn baby. To offset this, researchers recommend that women of childbearing age take a multivitamin containing 400 micrograms of folate every day if they are following a low-carb diet—the same amount that the U.S. Public Health Service has recommended since 1992.

Vision Problems

There have been a handful of case reports of patients losing some degree of vision while on low-carb diets, although none of them are recent. In one case, a Navy pilot and an aircraft mechanic, both assigned to the same tour of duty on an aircraft carrier, put themselves on low-carb diets in an attempt to lose weight. The thirty-three-year-old pilot ate mostly cheese, meat, eggs, fish, and some green vegetables;

he took no nutritional supplements. The thirty-six-year-old mechanic ate cheese, eggs, and red meat, plus an occasional slice of bread, and took a vitamin C supplement every day. Within a few months, both had lost a significant amount of weight, but both were having vision problems.

Returning from night-training exercises, the pilot had difficulty following the "meatball"—a red tracking light on the carrier deck, meant to help guide him to a safe landing. And the mechanic began having trouble walking around the ship at night because, he complained, the red lights used for illumination were too dim.

Both men were hospitalized for tests, and both turned out to have sizable blind spots in their peripheral vision. Each scored worse on routine vision exams than he had previously. The pilot could not distinguish between red and green on a color-blindness test, and the mechanic had an opaque line around each cornea that is usually found only in people who are much older. There was also a reduction of nerve fibers in one part of his eye. Both men were found to be thiamine-deficient and were placed on supplements; they also were told to resume eating a normal diet. Once they did, the pilot's vision cleared up completely within a few months. The mechanic's vision also improved significantly, but three years later, he still had tiny blind spots in his peripheral vision.

In another case, the same physician reported that two patients with epilepsy reported vision problems after being placed on ketogenic diets in an attempt to control their seizures. Tests determined that both had a condition called bilateral optical neuropathy, in which blood flow to the optic nerve is reduced. In both cases, this was traced to a thiamine deficiency related to the ketogenic diet; when they were placed on supplements, they regained normal vision. Reporting in the March 1979 issue of the *British Journal of Ophthalmology*, researchers suggested that the risk of optic nerve dysfunction could be minimized by making sure patients on ketogenic diets have the function of their optic nerves evaluated periodically and take vitamin B supplements.

"It seems evident that low-carbohydrate diets provide inadequate levels of thiamine for long-term maintenance of normal tissue function," reported the physicians who wrote up the cases. However, they also acknowledged that the vast majority of patients on such diets did not report vision problems. "It may be that only certain people are prone to develop pathological changes of the optic nerve, even when thiamine intake is abnormally low," they said. "Nevertheless, optic neuropathy resulting from thiamine deficiency appears to be a documented risk of living on a prolonged low-carbohydrate diet, and it is recommended that thiamine be given to patients on the [low-carb] dietary regime."

6.

The Business of
Low-Carb Lifestyles

Fans like to say that low-carb isn't a diet—it's a lifestyle. But make no mistake: It's also big business.

If you need proof of that, look no further than your grocery store. In the first nine months of 2004 alone, food manufacturers introduced 1,800 new products carrying labels that touted a low- or reduced-carbohydrate content—up from a mere 211 in all of 2001.

The products run the gamut—from pastas to waffle mix to tomato sauce and Fudgsicles. In the dairy aisle, some brands of milk and yogurt carry a large red-and-blue "A," indicating that they've been given the Atkins seal of approval, while the South Beach Diet has teamed up with Kraft to put its own seal of approval on 200 products, ranging from

Triscuits to fat-free Cool Whip and Philadelphia lite cream cheese. "Kraft is looking for ways to make weight management easier," the company's vice president of health and wellness said when announcing the deal.

Altruistic sentiments aside, there's little doubt that the company, like hundreds of others, is hoping to cash in on this hot dietary trend. And it's even making people who support the low-carb approach nervous. "I think it's going to sabotage low-carb diets," says Linda Stern, M.D., of the University of Pennsylvania Health Systems, who did two studies on low-carb diets in 2000 and 2001. At that time, there were very few low-carb prepared foods on the market, meaning that her patients had to make everything they ate from scratch—something that automatically made their diet far healthier than the one they had been eating. "That's why I couldn't even appreciate the controversy around low-carb diets," says Stern. "I was taking a population of patients who were incredibly unhealthy, who were eating donuts and bagels for breakfast and pizza and fries and burgers for lunch, and drinking a thousand calories and day and more in soda, and I was basically saying 'You're going to be eating vegetables and meat.' How could that be any worse than what they were already eating?"

But today, Stern's patients would be able to continue eating essentially the same diet they'd been eating before, thanks to all the new products that have flooded the marketplace: low-carb bagels and low-carb donuts; pizza with low-carb crust; fast-food hamburgers on low-carb buns. Even lower-carb french fries may soon join be available, thanks to a lower-carb potato that has been developed by a company in the Netherlands.

Many experts think the trend is taking a course that is unnervingly parallel to that of the low-fat trend of the past fifteen years, which was to try to sell food by insinuating that people could eat all they wanted of a particular product because it didn't contain fat. That's something that many experts believe had a lot to do with the failure of the low-fat message, and one that low-carb proponents are not eager to repeat.

"We have to decrease self-interest to encourage long-term behavioral trends," Dr. Fred Pescatore, M.D., author of the low-carb diet books *Thin for Good* and *The Hamptons Diet*, said in 2003 at a food industry meeting billed as the first LowCarBiz Summit. "We can't be like low-fat. We can't be a fad."

Marion Nestle, Ph.D., a professor of nutrition sciences at New York University, edited the 1988 Surgeon General's guidelines that helped to establish the eat-less-fat message. What it didn't say—but should have—she says now, is that calories also count. "We believed that if people reduced the amount of fat in their diets, they would automatically reduce the number of calories they were taking in," she says. "That was unbelievably naïve in retrospect, because what I never anticipated is how food companies would respond. And that response was to produce low-fat and no-fat products that are just as high in calories, which obviously isn't going to help anybody lose weight."

What makes this even more worrisome is the fact that the low-carb label is getting slapped on just about everything. "Even low-fat didn't manifest itself in the same way," says Suzanne Prong Eygabroat, director of information services at Productscan Online and Marketing Intelligence Service, which keeps the world's largest database of new product offerings.

"Yes, you would find low-fat [labels] on foods like yogurt or dairy or meat products that are traditionally high in fat. But with low-carb, they are taking products that are not very high in carbs to begin with and marketing them as low-carb."

They're also using marketing sleights of hand to make these products appeal to consumers. There are a number of low-carb peanut butters on the market, for instance, and if you check the nutrition labels, you'll see that they do indeed have a lower carb count—by exactly one gram. Another manufacturer is offering a roll that it calls the "wiser kaiser"—although if you look more closely, you'll find that it contains thirteen grams of carbohydrate, which isn't exactly low-carb in most dietitians' book—if that's even how many it has.

When KCBS in Los Angeles asked a lab to test a bagel billed as having fifteen grams of carbs, the lab reported that it actually had more than three times that many—fifty-five grams. And when *Dateline NBC* tested a number of items billed as "low-carb" on the menus of major restaurant chains, it found that these items, too, varied widely—sometimes from one shop to the next. For instance, *Dateline NBC* tested tested a chicken-and-cheese sandwich at a major sandwich shop in Manhattan; it claimed to have 8.5 grams of net carbs but in fact it had 45.11. On the other hand, the same item at another outlet in the same chain had the right amount of carbs, the program reported.

The Food and Drug Administration has said that in order to protect consumers, it plans to issue regulations defining just what makes a product low-carbohydrate, just as it set standards defining low-fat at the beginning of that trend. It's not clear when the regulations will come down, but manufacturers and trade associations are already lobbying: The Grocery Manufacturers of America suggests that products with less than 0.5 grams of carbohydrate per serving be labeled "carb-free," and those with less than 9 grams per serving be labeled "low-carb."

Even as it debates the new regulations, however, the FDA has been moving to curtail some of the low-carb labeling. It ordered Russell Stover to stop billing mint patties, toffee squares, and pecan delights as "low-carb," because they were no lower in carbs than comparable products, and told Peak Performance Foods, which makes sports snacks, to stop doing the same with its Peak Performance Pro-Bites.

Major food companies aren't the only businesses developing and/or marketing low-carb products. Many of the diet plans themselves are offering food products to help dieters comply. The Zone Diet sells energy bars, drink mixes, and nutritional supplements, as well as frozen meals ($8.95 for a two-pack) that adhere to the diet's 40:30:30 ratio of carbs to protein and fat, and which are available in flavors such as Chicken Dijon and Beef Jardiniere. The website for Pescatore's Hamptons Diet provides dieters with a link through which they can purchase macadamia nut oil, which the diet promotes heavily. And let's not forget Atkins Nutritionals, which sells everything from low-carb pita bread ($7.49 for two six-packs) to Atkins-trademarked Endulge chocolate bars, sale price $18.99 (down from $22.35) for a box of fifteen.

But Collette Heimowitz, director of education and research for Atkins Nutritionals, insists that there's a big difference in quality between the products that Atkins is distributing and those being marketed by major food manufacturers, who simply retool their ingredients just so they can slap a low-carb label on the resulting products.

"The integrity of some of these products that these food companies are coming out with is really lacking," she explains. "I mean, they have added sugars in them, the serving sizes are too small, they have trans-fats, sugar alcohols that give people diarrhea."

Heimowitz added that the Atkins company spends millions of dollars testing the "integrity" of its products to make sure that they don't cause increases in blood sugar or have other side effects.

Suzanna Eygabroat, whose job is observing product trends, says she gives Atkins a lot of credit. "Atkins is brilliant at the science of marketing low-carb," she says, noting that the company has stayed one step ahead of everyone else right from the start. Atkins began selling nutritional supplements by mail in 1989, and eight years later added a snack bar called the Atkins Advantage Bar, which comes in a variety of flavors, including chocolate and peanut butter. Then, in 2000, the company hired new managers to develop a much broader series of products to help people following the diet. Most recently, they licensed the Atkins name to a variety of products made by other companies, another move Eygabroat called "brilliant," since indications are that the market for low-carb foods may have reached a plateau.

But Heimowitz and Stuart Trager, M.D., the company's medical director, said the point behind all these things that the Atkins company has done is simply to make it easier for people to stay on the diet by helping them to identify low-carb foods. "We're doing it to make compliance easier," says Heimowitz. "They don't feel so restricted, it gives variety, it serves all those purposes to help dieters succeed."

Adds Trager, "This company's culture is one of doing the right thing, because doing the right thing is helping people."

But can the company really keep science and marketing separate, making sure that the former drives the latter, and not the other way around? Trager says he has no doubt that it can. "Atkins only survives if this approach works, if people have positive experiences," he says. "It doesn't do any good if more people do Atkins but don't get results."

The company announced in the fall of 2004 that it was teaming up with four major education groups, including the National Education Association and New York State United Teachers (a teachers' union), to provide educational materials on nutrition to schools. The company will help to pay for an NEA website for teachers and students, and will underwrite a publication on childhood obesity for state education policymakers.

The announcement was greeted with immediate howls of outrage from dietitians. "How can a group that says we should all stay away from peaches, bananas, pears, potatoes, rice—all the staples of our lives, and the ones kids like—turn around and say they're going to work with kids?" demands says Keith-Thomas Ayoob, Ph.D., an associate professor of pediatrics at Albert Einstein College of Medicine in New York City and a registered dietitian.

Ayoob was not alone in his outrage. The Partnership for Essential Nutrition, a coalition of consumer and nutrition groups announced a letter-writing campaign targeting the NEA and the teachers' union. In a statement, Barbara Moore, Ph.D., president of Shape Up America!, one of the lead groups in the coalition, said the company had no business anywhere near the classroom.

"The low-carb marketers of the Atkins diet are using a cunning strategy to place their name and logo in an arena that should be sacrosanct—our nation's schools," she said. "Although the stated goal is to combat childhood obesity, the real agenda is to continue to portray carbohydrates as the nutritional equivalent of snake oil and to target this information at vulnerable children."

But Trager says that the company's only goal is to help children make better nutritional choices—away from refined and processed carbohydrates and toward whole foods. "This isn't a case of us going into schools and pushing products," he says. "This isn't a case of us putting children on Atkins. This is a case of us going to educational organizations and saying 'How can we help?' "

Besides, he says, company officials will not be going into schools to do any teaching; rather, they'll be providing educational materials to the teachers.

"Because they're not teaching the kids directly, it's okay?" says Ayoob, noting that all the educational materials will undoubtedly have the Atkins logo on them. "They're teaching the teachers that are going to be teaching the kids! This is just another example of this company mortgaging the health of our kids for financial gain."

Says Trager, "I'm so sick of hearing that we're mortgaging the health of our kids. Obesity is a terrible public health epidemic. We want to do what we can to help."

Some analysts believe the low-carb trend has already peaked, at least as far as the marketplace is concerned. Indeed, there are signs that it is leveling off. "Some say retailers can't push their products out fast enough," she says. And the Atkins company itself announced a reorganization last fall.

But Eygabroat doesn't think the market for low-carb products is going to vanish anytime soon. While it's unlikely that companies will be introducing new low-carb products at the rate they have been, she says, "I think the carb attribute is going to weave its way into the fabric of new products for quite a long time."

How long? Eygabroat laughs. "Until someone who's sharper at marketing than Atkins can knock it off its pedestal."

When is a Carb Not a Carb?

Many of the new "carb-friendly" products on the market sport labels that proudly tout their low numbers of "net carbs." How valid this is, however, is a matter of debate. Although the FDA gives food manufacturers a formula by which to calculate the total carbohydrates in a product—a total that must be listed on the nutrition label—the manufacturers themselves came up with the term "net carbs" as a way of promoting their products to carbohydrate-conscious consumers. The theory behind these "net carbs"—or "impact carbs" as some manufacturers call them—is that not all carbohydrates are created equal. Some, such as sucrose and fructose, cause blood sugar to soar. Others, such as fiber, glycerin, and sugar alcohols, cause it to go up very little. Therefore, the manufacturers maintain, people who are counting carbs shouldn't have to worry about them. They subtract these carbs from the total carbs count and voila! Net carbs.

The FDA permits manufacturers to do this under an agreement hammered out in 2001. But many experts say that there are a couple of problems with this approach. First, many of these "lower-carb" products have as many calories as the regular-carb version, so their overall benefit to someone trying to lose weight is questionable.

Second, in the rush to make more carb-friendly products, manufacturers are removing blood-sugar-raising carbs such as flour and sugar from their products and replacing them with ingredients such as sugar alcohols, whose impact on the body isn't well understood. Although these ingredients have been used in small quantities in foods for some time, they're now being used in much larger amounts than before, with results that have yet to be determined. One thing we do know, however, is that sugar alcohols can have a laxative effect when ingested in large quantities.

7.

Is Low-Carb the Right Approach for You?

By now you should have a better understanding of some of the issues surrounding low-carb diets. You know that there are many concerns about their safety, but also some promising data. You also know that it will be years before we have answers to all the questions we have—and if you're like most people, you don't want to sit around for years waiting for them.

So how can you figure out if a low-carb diet is right for you now—and how do you proceed if you decide that it is? To find out, we turned to the people doing the research, and they suggested that you start by asking yourself the following questions.

- How much weight do you have to lose? "If you're thinking about doing this just to lose the five pounds to fit in your swimsuit, then I'd say this is probably not the best way to do it," says Duke University's Eric Westman, M.D. "But if you have a medical condition like obesity that's causing diabetes, that's causing high blood pressure, that you need to take medications to control, this might be something worth considering, because you're dealing with a problem that's serious," which might justify a more radical dietary approach.

- Have you tried and failed at a more conventional low-fat diet? If not, consider trying one of them first—we know more about their safety and long-term effects.

- What's your family's health history? Does it include problems that could be potentially be aggravated by a low-carb diet? If, for instance, there's a history of kidney problems in the family, that puts you at a higher-than-normal risk of developing them, too. So you might want to steer clear of a low-carb diet, because the higher protein intake can stress the kidneys.

If your mother and grandmother had osteoporosis, you'll need to consider the fact that some studies show an increased calcium loss for people on low-carb diets; if you choose to proceed, you'll at least need to take a supplement—keeping in mind that there's conflicting information as to whether supplements are effective.

• Is this something you'll be able to keep up for the long haul—a lifestyle as opposed to a diet? Or will you miss carbs so much that you're likely to cheat? The measure of success of any diet isn't how much weight you lose in the short term; it's how well you can keep it off, says Harvard's Walter Willett, M.D. "Pick a plan you think you can stick to in the long run," he says.

If you've evaluated all the risks and benefits and come to the conclusion that the low-carb approach is right for you, here's some advice from the experts. One word of caution: This book is meant to help you sort through all the claims and counterclaims that are being made about low-carb diets. It is not meant to take the place of your physician's advice, as the experts all stress in their first piece of advice below.

Consult with your doctor before doing anything. If you definition of cutting carbs is passing up the dinner rolls, you can probably skip this step. But if you're planning to do a full-fledged Atkins-style low-carb diet, you should talk to your doctor about it first, says Westman. That's because low-carb diets can have an extreme effect on your metabolism; you need to talk to your physician about the benefits and risks involved. "This diet has a much more powerful effect on the body than most others," says Westman. "And because of that, you need to do it under a doctor's supervision."

If you're taking medication for diabetes or high blood pressure, consider seeking out a physician with expertise treating people on low-carb diets. During the early weeks on a low-carb diet, you're likely to lose a lot of water weight; you'll also experience dramatic changes in your blood-sugar levels, says *Protein Power*'s Michael Eades. If you're taking diabetes and/or blood-pressure medications, they'll have to be adjusted—probably more than once. "If your medications aren't altered, you can have low blood sugar that can be dangerous; you can have low blood pressure that can be dangerous," explains Duke University's William Yancy. M.D. Physicians who don't have much experience working with patients on low-carb diets may have more trouble fine-tuning medications in response to the metabolic changes you're undergoing.

Have baseline blood tests taken, and get re-tested periodically during the course of the diet. "I would definitely recommend getting your blood checked first, because anytime you have a change in your nutrition intake, it can change your body metabolism," says Westman. "If it's not normal to begin with, you're probably going to have more side effects." It's particularly important to know your cholesterol and triglyceride levels before starting a low-carb diet, so you can judge how they respond to your new eating plan. Remember that one in every three or four low-carb dieters experiences an increase instead of a decrease in blood lipid levels; if you're one of them, you need to know about it so you can correct the problem, either by taking cholesterol-lowering drugs or by stopping the diet. As part of your initial workup, you might also consider having a kidney-function test done, to make sure you don't have any mild dysfunctions that would respond unfavorably to the increased protein levels you'll be consuming on a low-carb plan.

Skip the induction phase: Some low-carb diets

include an "induction phase" of one or more weeks, designed to jolt your body out of its dependence on carbs and switch it into fat-burning mode by going almost entirely cold turkey on carbs. Perhaps not surprisingly, this is when many of the side effects seem to occur, and many experts feel that these induction phases are unnecessarily hard on your body. "The main form of some of these diets, like the South Beach diet, are actually pretty good," says Willett. By skipping the induction phase, "You'll still lose weight—you might just lose it a little more slowly," he says, while getting the most nutritional benefits. "In the long run, you'll end up with the same weight loss," he says. "And I think the important part is finding the diet you can live with for the long run."

Take a multivitamin. Most low-carb diets are not very well balanced, nutritionally speaking, because when you cut out carb-laden foods like fruits and grains, you're also cutting out more than just carbs— you're cutting out all the other nutrients that come wrapped into that piece of fruit or bowl of oatmeal. Every doctor interviewed recommended that if you go on a low-carb diet, you make up for at least some of what you're missing by taking a multivitamin. Many of the plans suggest other supplements as well;

Eades, for instance, particularly likes to see his patients taking extra potassium and magnesium. If you've chosen a low-carb plan that recommends supplements, ask your doctor whether you should take them.

Consider working with a dietitian. "Anybody who's obese and wants to go on a diet should consider this," says Washington University's Samuel Klein, M.D. The dietitian can help you tweak your diet—low-carb or otherwise—to make it as healthy as possible, as well as help you develop a meal plan that fits both your diet and your lifestyle.

Choose lean meats and unsaturated fats wherever possible. For many people, the appeal of low-carb diets is the freedom to eat steak, bacon, cheese, etc.— in other words, the sorts of foods that are verboten in conventional diets. But most researchers agree that there's just too much evidence linking saturated fats to heart disease and cancer to recommend such a liberal approach. Rather, they suggest building the diet around chicken, fish, and other lean proteins. Even Atkins, who in the earliest editions of his book cheerfully told followers they could indulge in foods such as fried pork rinds and bacon and cheese soufflé, began to encourage them to choose leaner foods, such as turkey meatloaf and lean pork tenderloin, in the most recent edition of the book.

Be alert for side effects, particularly those that linger. Many people complain of side effects such as headache, fatigue, nausea, constipation, and muscle cramping when they begin a low-carb diet. These typically occur during the induction phase, and disappear within a couple weeks. If you've skipped the induction phase but still have side effects, or if they last longer than a couple weeks, they could be a sign that something more serious is wrong. Muscle cramping in particular is a red flag because it may indicate that your electrolytes are off-kilter, a problem you should take seriously, since it can lead to more serious problems such as heart arrhythmias. Consult your doctor if you experience any of these side effects.

Drink plenty of water and other fluids. Low-carb diets are believed to carry an increased risk of kidney stones. Drinking lots of water will help prevent them from forming. It will also help prevent the dehydration that often occurs during the early phases of low-carb diets. Some low-carb dieters say that drinking a cup or two of bouillon every day helps to prevent dehydration, and Yancy and Westman encourage their patients to consider doing this.

Eat the full allotted number of vegetables. Let's

face it, most people go on low-carb diets because they can eat butter and cheese—not because they can eat vegetables. But vegetables are some of the most nutrient-dense foods around. You're already eliminating a potential source of vitamins and minerals by cutting out fruits and other carbs. Now's not the time to skimp on your veggies.

Get a variety of vegetables and fruits; don't just eat the same ones over and over again. "Since each little plant has own unique profile of micronutrients, you can see that the wider variety you eat, the better off you are," says Eades. Be adventurous; try something new like prickly pears or tomatillos. If you look at the diets of our hunter-gatherer ancestors, you discover they ate about 150 different foods, he says, compared to the average American who (regardless of diet) eats something like twenty-five.

Exercise! Nearly every book on low-carb diets encourages followers to exercise. Atkins went so far as to call it "nonnegotiable," and all the doctors consulted agreed, as long as you are physically able to do so. (This is yet another reason to consult your doctor before starting to diet.) Exercise is an important part of any healthy lifestyle, whether or not you're on a low-carb diet. So if you're not in the habit of exercising, now's the time to start.

Go by the book. If you're not going to consult a doctor or dietitian, at least pick up one of the many low-carb diet books and read it thoroughly. All too often, people get their information from friends and the Internet, and end up with a hodgepodge of misconceptions, not to mention a piecemeal diet. Better to spring for the price of a paperback and get the real deal, including the theories behind the diet.

Re-evaluate periodically. We have data on the safety and effectiveness of low-carb diets for a year. But after that, it's anybody's guess. So how do you know whether to keep going? "Follow up with your doctor, and measure everything," advises Westman. By that he means weight loss, blood sugar, blood lipids, and all the other sorts of things that a physician normally measures during a physical exam—plus any that are specific to your personal risk factors, such as a bone-mineral density test to indicate whether osteoporosis is developing. "While these are not perfect measures, at least they will give you some way to monitor the safety of the diet," says Westman. In many ways, it's no different than an experimental drug that the FDA has approved for use for six months or a year. "If someone is happy with the results and wants to stay on it longer, it's really the doctor's judgment," Westman says.

Appendix

WEIGHT-LOSS ADVERTISING:
An Analysis of Current Trends
Richard L. Cleland
Walter C. Gross
Laura D. Koss
Matthew Daynard
Karen M. Muoio
Principal Authors
A REPORT OF THE STAFF
OF THE FEDERAL TRADE COMMISSION
September 2002

FEDERAL TRADE COMMISSION
TIMOTHY J. MURIS, *Chairman*
SHEILA F. ANTHONY, *Commissioner*
MOZELLE W. THOMPSON, *Commissioner*
ORSON SWINDLE, *Commissioner*
THOMAS B. LEARY, *Commissioner*

This report is a project of the staff of the Federal Trade Commission with the assistance of the Partnership for Healthy Weight Management, a coalition of representatives from science, academia, the health care profession, government, commercial enterprises, and organizations whose mission is to promote sound guidance on strategies for achieving and maintaining a healthy weight. The principal authors of this report are attorneys with the Bureau of Consumer Protection, Federal Trade Commission.

The views expressed in this report are those of the authors and do not necessarily represent the views of the Federal Trade Commission or any individual Commissioner. Special thanks are given to members of the Partnership, for their contributions to

Laura Muha

this report and to Michelle Rusk, an attorney with the Federal Trade Commission, for her assistance in editing this report, and Devenette Cox, who managed the data base for the report. The authors wish to acknowledge the contributions of Elizabeth Nichols, Eva Tayrose, Steve Sawchuk, Trisa Wilkens and Michelle Reeve for their assistance in the collection and coding of the advertisements reviewed in this report.

Full document with tables, illustrations, and footnotes may be viewed at http://www.ftc.gov/bcp/reports/weightloss.pdf.

Introduction

George L. Blackburn, M.D., Ph.D.

As health care professionals, we are concerned about the epidemic of obesity: the relations between excess body weight and such medical conditions as cardiovascular disease, hypertension, type 2 diabetes, osteoarthritis, sleep apnea, and certain cancers (such as breast, ovarian, prostate and colon) are well established. We are equally concerned about false and misleading claims in the advertising of weight loss products and services. Many promise immediate success without the need to reduce caloric intake or increase physical activity. The use of deceptive, false, or misleading claims in weight loss advertising is rampant and potentially dangerous. Many supplements, in particular, are of unproven value or have been linked to serious health risks.

A majority of adults in the United States are overweight or obese. All told, they invest over $30 billion a year in weight loss products and services. These consumers are entitled to accurate, reliable, and clearly-stated information on methods for weight management. They have a right to know if the weight loss products they're buying are helpful, useless, or even dangerous.

For this reason, the staff of the Bureau of Consumer Protection, Federal Trade Commission (FTC), joined with the Partnership for Healthy Weight Management—a coalition of representatives from science, academia, the health care professions, government agencies, commercial enterprises, and public interest organizations--to collect and analyze weight loss advertising. The Partnership's purpose is to promote sound guidance to the general public on strategies for achieving and maintaining a healthy weight. This report by the FTC staff is a major advance in that direction.

Evidence-based guidelines issued by the National Institutes of Health call for weight loss by simultaneously restricting caloric intake and increasing physical activity. Many studies demonstrate that obese adults can lose about 1 lb. per week and achieve a 5% to 15% weight loss by consuming 500 to 1,000 calories a day less than the caloric intake required for the maintenance of their current weight. Very low calorie diets result in faster weight loss, but lower rates of long-term success.

While exercise added to caloric restriction can help overweight and obese people achieve minimally faster weight loss early on, physical activity appears to be a very important treatment component for long-term maintenance of a reduced body weight. To lose weight and not regain it, ongoing changes in thinking, eating, and exercise are essential. Behavioral treatments that motivate therapeutic lifestyle changes can promote long-term success by helping obese individuals make necessary cognitive and lifestyle changes.

The public often perceives weight losses of 5% to 15% as small and insufficient even though they suffice to prevent and improve many of the medical problems associated with weight gain, overeating, and a sedentary lifestyle. Many in the weight loss industry promise effortless, fast weight loss, then support this misperception by bombarding Americans with spurious advertising messages touting physiologically impossible weight loss outcomes from the use of unproven products and services. All advertisers, whatever their choice of media--cable television, infomercials, radio, magazines, newspapers, supermarket tabloids, direct mail, or commercial e-mail and Internet websites--know that only those products and services that help people adopt lifestyles that balance caloric intake with caloric output will prevent and treat the disease of obesity.

KILLER DIETS

For certain businesses (weight loss franchises, pharmaceutical firms, food companies, the dietbook industry, makers of exercise equipment, suppliers of dietary supplements, to name a few) these deceptive and misleading advertisements prevent the public from hearing their messages, words that promote therapeutic lifestyle changes as advocated by professional societies and the U.S. Department of Health and Human Services. Data indicate that at any given time, almost 70 million Americans are trying to lose weight or prevent weight gain. In 2000 they spent approximately $35 billion on products they were told would help them achieve those objectives--videos, tapes, books, medications, foods for special dietary purpose, dietary supplements, medical treatments, and other related goods and services.

As with cigarette smoking and alcohol abuse, false or deceptive advertising of weight loss products and services puts people at risk. Many of the products and programs most heavily advertised are at best unproven and at worst unsafe. By promoting unrealistic expectations and false hopes, they doom current weight loss efforts to failure, and make future attempts less likely to succeed. In the absence of laws and regulations to protect the public against dangerous or misleading products, a priority exists for the media to willingly ascribe to the highest advertising standards, i.e., those that reject the creation and acceptance of advertisements that contain false or misleading weight loss claims.

The public would be well served by becoming more knowledgeable about the evidencebased guidelines, the scientifically-proven and medically-safe standards that underlie national public health policy. When more people know what's important and realistic in achieving and maintaining a healthy body weight, fewer will be inclined to waste their money, time, and effort on dangerous fads or miracle cures. The staff of the FTC's Bureau of Consumer Protection has provided an analysis of current trends in weight loss advertising. It is now up to the consumer and media to act in the best interest of the public health.

Laura Muha

George L. Blackburn, M.D., Ph.D.
S. Daniel Abraham Chair in Nutrition Medicine
Harvard Medical School, Boston, MA
Past President of The American Society for Clinical Nutrition,
North American Association for the Study of Obesity, and the
American Society for Parenteral and Enteral Nutrition

Executive Summary

This report attempts to take a comprehensive look at weight loss advertising. The need to do so is compelling. In the last decade, the number of FTC law enforcement cases involving weight loss products or services equaled those filed in the previous seven decades. Consumers spend billions of dollars a year on weight loss products and services, money wasted if spent on worthless remedies. This report highlights the scope of the problem facing consumers as they consider the thousands of purported remedies on the market, as well as the serious challenge facing law enforcement agencies attempting to prevent deceptive advertising.

According to the U.S. Surgeon General, overweight and obesity have reached epidemic proportions, afflicting 6 out of every 10 Americans. Overweight and obesity constitute the second leading cause of preventable death, after smoking, resulting in an estimated 300,000 deaths per year. The costs, direct and indirect, associated with overweight and obesity are estimated to exceed $100 billion a year.

At the same time, survey data suggest that millions of Americans are trying to lose weight.

The marketplace has responded with a proliferating array of products and services, many promising miraculous, quick-fix remedies. Tens of millions of consumers have turned to over-the-counter remedies, spending billions of dollars on products and services that purport to promote weight loss.

In the end, these quick-fixes do nothing to address the nation's or the individual's weight problem, and, if anything, may contribute to an already serious health crisis.

Once the province of supermarket tabloids and the back sections of certain magazines, over-the-top weight loss advertisements promising quick, easy weight loss are now pervasive in almost all media forms. At least that is the impression. But are the obviously deceptive advertisements really as widespread as they might appear watching late night television or leafing through magazines at the local newsstand? To answer this and other questions, we collected and analyzed a nonrandom sample of 300 advertisements, mostly disseminated during the first half of 2001, from broadcast and cable television, infomercials, radio, magazines, newspapers, supermarket tabloids, direct mail, commercial e-mail (spam), and Internet websites. In addition, to evaluate how weight-loss advertising has changed over the past decade, we collected ads disseminated in 1992 in eight national magazines to compare with ads appearing in 2001 in the same publications.

We conclude that false or misleading claims are common in weight-loss advertising, and, based on our comparison of 1992 magazine ads with magazines ads for 2001, the number of products and the amount of advertising, much of it deceptive, appears to have increased dramatically over the last decade.

Of particular concern in ads in 2001 are grossly exaggerated or clearly unsubstantiated performance claims. Although we did not evaluate the substantiation for specific products and advertising claims as part of this report, many of the claims we reviewed are so contrary to existing scientific evidence, or so clearly unsupported by the available evidence, that there is little doubt that they are false or deceptive. In addition to the obviously false claims, many other advertisements contain claims that appear likely to be misleading or unsubstantiated.

Falling into the too-good-to-be-true category are claims that: the user can lose a pound a day or more over extended periods of time; that substantial weight loss (without surgery) can be achieved without diet or exercise; and that users can lose weight regardless of how much they eat.

Also falling into this category are claims that a diet pill can cause weight loss in selective parts of the body or block absorption of all fat in the diet. These types of claims are simply inconsistent with existing scientific knowledge.

This report catalogues the most common marketing techniques used in 300 weight loss advertisements. Nearly all of the ads reviewed used at least one and sometimes several of the following techniques, many of which should raise red flags about the veracity of the claims.

Consumer Testimonials; Before/After Photos.

The headline proclaimed: "I lost 46 lbs in 30 days." Another blared, "How I lost 54 pounds without dieting or medication in less than 6 weeks!" The use of consumer testimonials is pervasive in weight-loss advertising. One hundred and ninety-five (65%) of the advertisements in the sample used consumer testimonials and 42% contained before-and-after pictures. These testimonials and photos rarely portrayed realistic weight loss. The average for the largest amount of weight loss reported in each of the 195 advertisements was 71 pounds. Fifty-seven ads reported weight loss exceeding 70 pounds, and 38 ads reported weight loss exceeding 100 pounds. The advertised weight loss ranges are, in all likelihood, simply not achievable for the products being promoted. Thirty-six ads used 71 different testimonials claiming weight loss of nearly a pound a day for time periods of 13 days or more.

Rapid Weight-loss Claims.

Rapid weight-loss claims were made in 57% of the advertisements in the sample. In some cases, the falsity of such claims is obvious, as in the ad that claimed that users could lose up to 8 to 10 pounds per week while using the advertised product.

No Diet or Exercise Required.

Despite the well-accepted prescription of diet and exercise for successful weight management, 42% of all of the ads reviewed promote an array of quick-fix pills, patches, potions, and programs for effortless weight loss and 64% of those ads also promised fast results. The ads claim that results can be achieved without reducing caloric intake or increasing physical activity. Some even go so far as to tell consumers "you can eat as much as you want and still lose weight."

Long-term/Permanent Weight-loss Claims.

"Take it off and keep it off" (longterm/permanent weight loss) claims were used in 41% of the ads in the sample. In fact, the publicly available scientific research contains very little that would substantiate long-term or permanent weight-loss claims for most of today's popular diet products. Accordingly, long-term or permanent weight-loss claims are inherently suspect.

Clinically Proven/Doctor Approved Claims.

Clinically proven and doctor approved claims are also fairly common in weight-loss advertisements, the former occurring in 40% and the latter in 25% of the ads in the sample. Some of the specific claims are virtually meaningless. For example, a representation such as, "Clinical studies show people lost 300% more weight even without dieting," may cause consumers to conclude mistakenly that the clinically proven benefits are substantial, whereas, in fact, the difference between use of the product and dieting alone could be quite small (1.5 lbs. vs. .5 lbs.). These claims do little to inform consumers and most ads fail to provide consumers with sufficient information to allow them to verify the advertisers' representations. Moreover, the Federal Trade Commission, in past law enforcement actions, has evaluated the available scientific evidence for many of the ingredients expressly advertised as clinically proven, and challenged the weight-loss efficacy claims for these ingredients.

Natural/Safe Weight-loss Claims.

Safety claims are also prevalent in weight-loss advertising. Nearly half of all the ads in the sample (42%) contained specific claims that the advertised products or services are safe and 71% of those ads also claimed that the products were "all natural." Safety claims can be difficult to evaluate, especially when so many ads fail to disclose the active ingredients in the product. On the other hand, some advertisements disclose ingredients, e.g., ephedra alkaloids, that make unqualified safety claims misleading. Nevertheless, marketers in almost half (48%) of the ads that identified ephedra as a product ingredient made safety claims. Only 30% of the ads that identified ephedra as an ingredient included a specific health warning about its potential adverse effects.

Historical Comparison.

To develop a perspective on how weight-loss advertising has changed over time, this report also compares advertisements appearing in a sample of magazines published in 2001 with ads in the same magazines in 1992. Compared to 1992, readers in 2001 saw more diet ads, more often, and for more products. Specifically,

- The frequency of weight-loss advertisements in these magazines more than doubled,

and

- The number of separate and distinct advertisements tripled.

Moreover, the type of weight-loss products and services advertised dramatically shifted from "meal replacements" (57%), in 1992 to dietary supplements (66%), in 2001. Meal replacement products typically facilitate the reduction of caloric intake by replacing high-calorie foods with lower-calorie substitutes, whereas dietary supplements are commonly marketed (55%) with claims that reducing caloric intake or increasing physical activity is unnecessary.

The considerable changes in the methods used to promote weight-loss products are the most revealing indication of the downward spiral to deception in weight-loss advertising. The 2001 advertisements were much more likely than the 1992 ads to use dramatic consumer testimonials and before-and-after photos, promise permanent weight loss, guarantee weight-loss success, claim that weight loss can be achieved without diet or exercise, claim that results can be achieved quickly, claim that the product is all natural, and make express or implied claims that the product is safe.

Finally, although both the 1992 and 2001 examples include unobjectionable representations, as well as almost certainly false claims, the 2001 advertisements appear much more likely to make specific performance promises that are misleading.

Conclusion.

The use of false or misleading claims in weight-loss advertising is rampant.

Nearly 40% of the ads in our sample made at least one representation that almost certainly is false and 55% of the ads made at least one representation that is very likely to be false or, at the very least, lacks adequate substantiation. The proliferation of such ads has proceeded in the face of, and in spite of, an unprecedented level of FTC enforcement activity, including the filing of more than 80 cases during the last decade. The need for critical evaluation seems readily apparent. Government agencies with oversight over weight-loss advertising must continually reassess the effectiveness of enforcement and consumer and business education strategies. Trade associations and selfregulatory groups must do a better job of educating their members about standards for truthful advertising and enforcing those standards. The media must be encouraged to adopt meaningful clearance standards that weed out facially deceptive or misleading weight-loss claims. The past efforts of the FTC and the others to encourage the adoption of media screening standards have been largely unsuccessful. Nevertheless, as this report demonstrates, the adoption and enforcement of standards would reduce the amount of blatantly deceptive advertising disseminated to consumers and efforts to encourage the adoption of such standards should continue. Finally, individual consumers must become more knowledgeable about the importance of achieving and maintaining healthy weight, more informed about how to shop for weight-loss products and services, and more skeptical of ads promising quick-fixes.

I. An Overview
A. A Never-Ending Quest for Easy Solutions

Since at least 1900, American consumers have been searching for a safe and effective way to lose weight. As a nation, it has been a losing battle. Overweight and obesity have reached epidemic proportions.[1] An estimated 61 percent of U.S. adults are overweight or obese, and the trend is in the wrong direction.[2] Overweight and obesity constitute the second leading cause of preventable death, after smoking, resulting in an estimated 300,000 deaths per year at a cost (direct and indirect) that exceeds $100 billion a year.[3]

The struggle to shed unwanted pounds usually resolves itself into choosing between responsible products or programs that offer methods for achieving moderate weight loss over time and "miracle" products or services that promise fast and easy weight loss without sacrifice. Over the course of the last century, popular weight-loss methods have included: prescription and over-the-counter drugs and dietary supplements; surgical procedures such as gastro-intestinal bypass surgery, gastroplasty (stomach stapling), and jaw wiring; the television shows of motivational weightloss gurus; commercial weight-loss centers; commercial diet drinks; doctor-supervised very-lowcalorie diets, complete with their own vitamin shots, fiber cookies, and drinks; the development of fat-free, low-fat, fake-fat, and sugar-free foods; weight-loss support groups; exercise trends such as aerobics and body building; and cellulite creams.

Almost all weight-loss experts agree that the key to long-term weight management lies in permanent lifestyle changes that include, among other things, a nutritious diet at a moderate caloric level and regular physical exercise. Nevertheless, advertisements for weight-loss products and services saturate the marketplace, with many promising instantaneous success without the need to reduce caloric intake or increase physical activity.

This is not a new phenomenon. In the last 100 years, various types of weight loss products and programs have gained and lost popularity, ranging from the ludicrous – diet bath powders, soaps, and shoe inserts – to the dangerous, such as the fen/phen diet pill combination.[4] Around the 1900s, popular weight-loss drugs included animal-derived thyroid, laxatives, and the poisons arsenic and strychnine; eventually each was shown to cause weight loss only temporarily, and usually to be unsafe to use. In the 1930s, doctors prescribed dinitrophenol, a synthetic insecticide and herbicide that increases human metabolism so drastically that organs fail, causing blindness and other health problems. The hormone human chorionic gonadotropin (HCG) became popular in the 1950s for weight loss, and resurfaced recently, even though the FDA exposed it decades ago as effective only to treat Fröhlich's Syndrome, a particular genetic imbalance occurring only in boys.[5]

The 1990s saw an explosion in dietary supplement marketing, many of which are of unproven value and/or have been linked to serious health risks.[6] As discussed in this report, the Federal Trade Commission has brought numerous cases against the advertisers of weight-loss supplements for making false or misleading advertising claims. Other products may raise serious safety concerns. For example, experts, including the American Medical Association, have raised concerns about the safety of ephedra, a popular diet pill ingredient,[7] and Health Canada recently warned Canadian citizens against using ephedra for dieting because of its dangerous propensities.[8]

B. The Role of Advertising for Weight-loss Products and Services
As noted above, consumers may choose from a myriad of weight-loss products and services. Consumers make their selections based, in part, on advertising. Advertising that presents false or misleading information may distort consumer

decision making. Even more troubling, if the entire field of weight-loss advertising is subject to wide-spread deception, then advertising loses its important role in the efficient allocation of resources in a free-market economy. If the purveyors of the "fast and easy fixes" drive the marketplace, then others may feel compelled to follow suit or risk losing market share to the hucksters who promise the impossible. Public health suffers as well. The deceptive promotion of quick and easy weight-loss solutions potentially fuels unrealistic expectations on the part of consumers. Consumers who believe that it is really possible to lose a pound a day may quickly lose interest in losing a pound or less a week.

C. Weight Loss: A Multi-Billion Dollar Industry

More than two thirds of American adults are trying either to lose weight or to forestall weight gain, according to a 1996 survey of 107,000 people by the Centers for Disease Control and Prevention ("CDC").[9] The nearly 29 percent of men and 44 percent of women who are trying to lose weight[10] (an estimated 68 million American adults) comprise a huge potential market for sellers of weight-loss products and services. No wonder overall sales in the weight-loss/weight-control industry are burgeoning. According to an article in the Atlanta Business Chronicle, consumers spent an estimated $34.7 billion in 2000 on weight-loss products and programs.[11] This figure includes sales of books, videos, and tapes, low-calorie foods and drinks, sugar substitutes, meal replacements, prescription drugs, over-the-counter drugs, dietary supplements, medical treatments, commercial weight-loss chains, and other products or services related to weight-loss or weightmaintenance. Although total sales information is not available, the figures that are available are impressively large. For example, year 2000 sales for the eight largest weight-loss chains totaled $788 million, and sales for dietary supplements that purport to promote weight loss accounted for $279 million in retail outlets alone.[12] In a report from the Business Communications Company based on 1999 figures, total sales for weight-loss supplements were estimated at $4.6 billion.[13] This corresponds with estimates from the CDC, based on a five-state random-digit telephone survey, that 7% of the adult population used one or more non-prescription weight-loss products during 1996 through 1998.[14] The authors extrapolate from this survey that an estimated 17.2 million Americans used nonprescription weight-loss products during this time period.[15]

The amount of total sales for unproven or worthless products is not known, but it is substantial. Infomercials, direct mail advertising, and free-standing inserts can generate tens of millions of dollars in sales within a short period of time for a single product, and, as this report demonstrates, there are hundreds, perhaps even thousands, of weight-loss products on the market. These forms of saturation advertising do not require high response rates to be highly profitable. As an example of the prevalence of hard-sell marketing for non-prescription weight-loss products, spending on infomercials (usually 30-minute to an hour programs pitching products for direct sale via telephone call-ins) for weight-loss and nutrition products exceeded $107 million in 1999.[16] The alarming increase in overweight and obesity combined with marketers' easy access to mass media outlets makes the business of weight loss a booming enterprise.

II. Collection Methodology and Coding

This report looks at weight-loss advertising disseminated through broadcast and cable television, infomercials, radio, magazines, newspapers (including free-standing inserts in Sunday newspapers), supermarket tabloids, direct mail, commercial e-mail (spam), and Internet websites. We collected a total of 300 advertisements from a variety of sources. Except as noted with regard to Internet sites, we did not attempt to select a scientifically random sample.[17] At the same time, no effort was made to collect just "bad" ads. In general, these advertisements appeared between February and May 2001.

Television and radio advertisements: Members of the

Partnership for Healthy Weight Management18 (the Partnership) monitored television and radio advertisements and sent identifying information to the FTC staff, who ordered copies of the ads from Video Monitoring Service. Twenty radio and television ads were included in our sample.

Infomercials: The FTC staff obtained a list of twenty-eight infomercials appearing between January 1, 2001 and May 7, 2001 from Infomercial Monitoring Service, Inc. and ordered six infomercials, based on the product description and the date the infomercial initially aired. We gave preference to infomercials that appeared to involve relatively new products and excluded infomercials marketing exercise equipment and electronic devices. When there were two infomercials for the same product, we selected the infomercial with the most recent initial appearance date.19

Magazines and supermarket tabloids: The FTC staff selected the following magazines and supermarket tabloids for monitoring: *Cosmopolitan*, *Family Circle*, *Fitness*, *First for women*, *Glamour*, *Globe*, *Ladies Home Journal*, *Let's Live*, *Marie Claire*, *McCalls*, *National Enquirer*, *National Examiner*, *Redbook*, *Rosie*, *Self*, *Soap Opera Digest*, *Star*, *Sun*, *Weekly World News*, *Woman's Day*, *Women's Fitness*, and *Women's Own*. We selected some of the publications because of their past history of running questionable weight loss advertisements. With regard to magazines published on a monthly basis, we reviewed each issue from February through May for weight-loss advertisements. We reviewed only selected editions of weekly publications.

Newspapers: The FTC staff obtained a sample of U.S. newspaper advertisements from Burrelle's Information Services, a newspaper clipping service. The ads appeared during April and the first week of May 2001. We included newspaper ads in our sample if they contained references to specific amounts of weight loss, e.g., lose 30 pounds by summer, or John Doe lost 30 pounds.

Direct Mail and Unsolicited Commercial e-mail (spam): We collected direct mail and spam ads from the FTC staff, members of the Partnership, and consumers.

Internet Ads: The Partnership and two Northern Illinois University researchers organized a "surf day" project to identify relevant websites. In December 2000, a student-team collected data, using 14 popular search engines and 139 keyword search terms, about Internet websites containing weight-loss related information.20 Through this process, participants located thousands of Internet websites. Researchers compiled URL and other information about the websites in a database. The FTC staff randomly selected every 50th still-active site in the database until it had accumulated a representative sample of 44 commercial sites that promoted weight-loss products and/or services.

The FTC staff collected and coded the following information from each advertisement: company name; product name; product type, e.g., meal replacement; publication and publication dates; method of dissemination (broadcast TV, cable TV, infomercial, radio, magazine, newspaper, tabloid, direct mail, free standing insert, unsolicited commercial e-mail (spam), and Internet website); and purchase options (retail outlet, website, direct mail, telephone, other). The FTC staff also coded the use of the following specific types of claims or advertising techniques: consumer testimonials; before-and-after photos; rapid weight-loss claims; lose weight without diet or exercise claims; long-term or permanent weight-loss claims; representations that the user will not fail no matter how many times he or she has failed before; clinically or scientifically proven claims; endorsements by medical professionals; money-back guarantees; and all-natural and/or safe claims. The FTC staff also recorded the specific text of the headline and representative claims for analysis.

We collected additional information from ads using consumer testimonials, including: the number of testimonials used; the high and low range of weight loss claimed, e.g., 10 lbs. in two weeks/30 lbs. in 30 days; whether there was a disclaimer associated with the use of the testimonials, what the disclaimer said, and whether the disclaimer was conspicuous.

With regard to safety, we collected information on whether potential side effects were disclosed. Where there was a safety warning, we recorded the text of the warning. The FTC staff collected information concerning the active ingredients in the product if the advertisement provided that information.

III. Analysis of Weight-loss Advertisements
A. General Observations

An ad for a product made from ground-up shells of shrimps, crabs, and lobsters claims, "Scientists dedicated years of research to come up with a high powered diet ingredient with no side effects" and asks, "Have you ever seen an overweight fish? Or an oyster with a few pounds too many? Everyone knows that sea animals never get fat." A testimonial in this ad alludes to the product's ability to select only unwanted fat deposits: "The best thing about [the product] is that my waist size is 3 inches smaller, now only 26 inches. And it has taken off quite some inches from my butts [sic] (5 inches) and thighs (4 inches), my hips now measure only 35 inches. I still wear the same bra size though. The fat has disappeared from exactly the right places." In fact, there is no convincing evidence that the shells of shrimps, crabs, or lobsters cause weight loss or that weight loss can be selectively targeted to specific parts of the body. An ad for a second product whose active ingredient is apple pectin is headlined, "LOSE UP TO 2 POUNDS DAILY... WITHOUT DIET OR EXERCISE! I LOST 44 POUNDS IN 30 DAYS!" The ad further claims that "Apple pectin is an energized enzyme that can ingest up to 900 times its own weight in fat. That's why it's a fantastic fat blocker." The ad claims that the product can "eliminate fat for effortless weight loss" and that it produces the "same results as jogging 10 miles per week, an hour of aerobics per day, 15 hours of cycling or swimming per week." In fact, there is no known pill that will cause up to two pounds of weight loss daily (with or without diet and exercise), and the claim of 44 pounds of weight loss in 30 days is not credible.

148

In an infomercial for yet another weight-loss product, a beaming spokesperson and a purported scientific expert standing in front of a colorful pastry display assure viewers that to lose weight while using the product, "you don't really need any willpower. You don't have to diet or deprive yourself of foods in any way." As the endorsers make these claims, the words "Call Now" and "Risk Free," with the telephone number to order, appear in large, yellow text on one part of the screen on a blue background. At the same time, dim and indistinct white letters on a moving, mottled background advise, "A healthy diet and exercise are required to lose weight."

The world of weight-loss advertising is a virtual fantasy land where pounds "melt away" while "you continue to eat your favorite foods"; "amazing pills . . . seek and destroy enemy fat"; researchers at a German university discover the "amazing weight loss properties" of asparagus; and the weight-loss efficacy of another product is comparable to "running a 20 mile marathon while you sleep." It's a world where, in spite of prevailing scientific opinion, no sacrifice is required to lose weight ("You don't change your eating habits and still lose weight"). Quick results are the (promised) norm ("The diet works three times faster than FASTING itself!"). You can learn how to lose weight with "No exercise. No drugs. No pills. And eat as much as you want – the more you eat, the more you lose." There is no need to worry because the products are "safe," "risk free,"and/or "natural," and some marketers are so concerned for your safety that they warn you to cut back if you lose too much weight ("If you begin to lose weight too quickly, take a few days off!!!"). You can always get your money back because so many of these "amazing" products are "guaranteed" (". . .we'll give you your money back. Straight away. No questions asked").

And for those who remain skeptical, there is an answer. The products are backed by "clinical studies" or are "clinically tested" ("Clinical and laboratory tests at leading universities and hospitals, have proven that this product is effective"). Even if they do not purport to be clinically proven, many claim to be the product of years of scientific research ("Scientists dedicated years of research to come up with a high powered diet ingredient with no side effects") or are "doctor recommended."

Moreover, according to many of the ads, you can "stay slim forever" because the weight loss is "permanent" ("I can still eat whatever I want without any danger of gaining the weight back."). Finally, you can say good-bye to the failure syndrome because no matter how many times you've tried to lose weight in the past, the product will give you the "secret to lasting weight loss success."

B. Media and Product Types

Three hundred advertisements for 218 different products or services were collected and reviewed. A list of the products is included in Appendix A. Table 1 identifies the number of ads for each type of medium.[21]

The advertisements covered virtually every kind of product or service imaginable. Categories with 10 or more advertisements included: dietary supplements (157), meal replacements (e.g., diet shakes) (33), hypnosis (27), food (15), diet plans/programs/diet centers (21), transdermal products (patches and creams) (11), and wraps (10). Some ads promoted multiple products, and in some instances, it was not possible to determine the product category based solely on the advertisement. Only about half (49%) of the advertisements for dietary supplement or transdermal products disclosed the product's active ingredients in the advertisement. Of those that identified ingredients, the most common were ephedra, chitosan, and chromium.[22]

C. Claims by Category

A clear pattern of claims and techniques emerged from our analysis. Nearly all of the ads reviewed used at least one and sometimes several of these techniques. Figure 1 shows the frequency of common advertising claims and techniques and what percentage of the 300 ads used the claim or technique. A composite ad showing the frequency of each claim or technique appears on page 8 of this report. Table 2 shows the percentage of ads by product category that contains the claims. The following sections discuss specific claims and techniques in detail.

I. Consumer Testimonials

Consumer testimonials are pervasive in weight-loss advertising. Of the advertisements in the sample, 195 (65%) used consumer testimonials as a mechanism to promote the weight-loss product or service. The ads that used this technique contained about five testimonials on average, with some containing as many as 50 or more. Testimonials were most often used in ads promoting hypnosis.

Testimonials rarely described modest or realistic successes, instead touting extraordinary and rapid weight loss. Nearly 90% of ads using consumer testimonials claimed specific amounts of weight loss and more than half (56%) included a specific time period for the largest amount of weight loss reported in the ad, e.g., "I lost 30 pounds in 30 days." The average for the largest amount of weight loss reported in each of the 195 advertisements was about 71 pounds. Fiftyseven (57) ads (30%) reported weight loss exceeding 70 pounds, and 38 ads (20%) reported weight loss exceeding 100 pounds.

In many instances ads used testimonials reporting weight loss in ranges that are, in all likelihood, simply not achievable for the products being promoted. Thirty-six ads used 71 different testimonials claiming weight loss of nearly a pound a day for time periods of 13 days or more. These ranged from claims of 22 pounds in 13 days to 120 pounds in seven weeks. All but three of these ads were for dietary supplement products.

There are many examples of implausible testimonials but perhaps the most remarkable is this one from a woman who claimed:

> 7 weeks ago I weighed 268 lbs, now I am down to just
> 148 lbs! During this time I didn't change my eating habits
> at all: the pounds must have disappeared only due to the

new slimming capsule. My appearance is so different that
my friends actually believe that I had liposuction.

The product featured in this advertisement claims to work
by preventing the absorption of fat in the digestive system. In
fact, weight loss of this magnitude would require a net calorie
deficit of 8,571 calories per day over the course of seven weeks.
Even complete fasting would not produce this kind of result.
Nevertheless, this testimonial was disseminated to millions of
Americans through *Cosmopolitan*, *Soap Opera Digest*, *National
Enquirer*, *Women's Day*, *Let's Live*, *Women's Own*, *McCall's*,
Star, and *First for women*.

Testimonials in weight-loss advertisements appear to serve
at least two functions. First, they convey an efficacy claim, i.e.,
the product works; and second, they attempt to minimize
consumer skepticism. Many potential purchasers of weight-loss
products have purchased other weight-loss products that failed.
The challenge for the advertiser is to convince the purchaser that
its product will work when all the others have not. One way to
do that is to present the purchaser with examples of "real
people" just like themselves who have used the product
successfully. Indeed, in some instances, particularly infomercials,
the endorser directly addresses viewers to reassure them that the
product really worked when all other products and programs
failed.

Weight-loss testimonials convey more than a limited
message about one person's experience. They also convey a very
convincing claim to consumers that the product is effective and,
in some instances, that the product will enable the user to
experience similarly dramatic results. Thus, testimonials can be
deceptive in at least three distinct ways. First, the testimonialist
may not have experienced the reported result. Testimonials that
claim that users lost more than 30 pounds in as little as 30 days
likely fall into this category. Second, the reported weight loss
may not be attributable to the product, but to other diet,
exercise, or lifestyle changes. Third, an advertisement presenting
testimonials claiming extreme and atypical weight loss as typical

or ordinary experiences is likely to be deceptive without an indication of the more modest weight loss results that the typical user would experience using the product.[23]

Typicality Disclaimers: The most common way to address this last issue is through disclaimers. Seventy (70) of the 195 ads (36%) had some form of disclaimer addressing the issue of whether the reported results are meant to be representative of users of the product or service. In only 18 of the cases, however, was the disclaimer conspicuous or proximate to the testimonials. In the vast majority of advertisements, disclaimers were buried in fine print footnotes or, in video ads, flashed as a video superscript too quickly for viewers to read. Table 3 provides a sample of disclaimers found in the selected advertisements.

Some of these disclaimers do little to inform consumers that the results reported in the advertisements are, at best, extreme cases, and that consumers should not expect to achieve similar results. For example, a disclaimer telling consumers that "results may vary" tells consumers almost nothing other than that everyone will not achieve 50 pounds of weight loss. With one or two notable exceptions, advertisers made no effort to provide specific information about the actual weight loss the average consumer could expect using a particular product.

2. Before/After Photos

Before-and-after photos, often appearing with testimonials, are commonly used in weight loss ads. Fortytwo percent (42%) of the ads in this sample contained before-and-after pictures. More than just graphic consumer testimonials, these pictures try to create an image of what the consumers could accomplish personally if they only used the advertised product. Before-and-after pictures usually fall into one of two categories: (1) the illustrated personal testimonial, and (2) the clinical comparison of isolated body portions.[24] The former type often contains the following elements:

Before Picture: Snapshot quality photograph of the subject that incorporates poor posture, neutral facial expression, unkempt hair, unfashionable attire, poor lighting, and washed out skin tones.

After Picture: Brightly lit (sometimes studio portrait quality) pose of smiling subject in fashionable, often skimpy, attire, shoulders held back, tummy tucked in, with a stylish hair style and carefully applied makeup.

Eighty-eight percent (88%) of the ads with before-and-after pictures contained illustrated testimonials. In television spots and infomercials, this type of before-and-after treatment often incorporates a before photograph superimposed over a videotaped segment featuring the subject after using the advertised product or service making his/her videotaped testimonial.

Another form of before-and-after illustration isolates one portion of a subject's anatomy, usually the waist or buttocks, to show purported results, sometimes in a progression of three or more photographs over a period of time. These pictures often emulate the kind of illustrations found in medical articles. A few ads (two in this sample) feature both types of before-and-after pictures. Eleven percent (11%) of the ads with before- and-after pictures featured "clinical" comparison pictures.

Often the only discernable difference in the before picture and the after picture is a change in posture and body control. In the before picture the subject's shoulders are slumped, the abdominal muscles are relaxed, and the pelvis thrust forward to emphasize body fat. The after picture shows the subject holding in his/her abdomen and/or holding back his/her shoulders to emphasize lean body mass. A close examination of the before picture in this type of ad raises the question of whether the subject needed to lose weight and suggests that little or no weight was actually lost.

Some before-and-after photographs clearly appear to have been altered, usually by placing an image of the after subject's head on the photographic image of another (very obese) subject's body. Finally, it is not always clear whether "clinical" before-and-after pictures are depicting the results from actual users of the advertised product or service or are intended merely to be illustrative of the product's or service's capacity to produce weight loss.

3. Rapid Weight-loss Claims

Fifty-seven percent (57%) of the ads in our sample promised rapid weight loss, often claiming that excess weight or fat can disappear in a matter of days or weeks. Claims in this category range from explicit promises of rapid weight loss ("A Quick Weight Loss Plan For People In A Hurry" "RAPID WEIGHT LOSS IN 28 DAYS!" "Clinically proven to help you lose weight . . . fast") through claims for immediate or near immediate results ("Starts to work within minutes" "Works in one minute" "You only have to stay on it 2 DAYS TO SEE RESULTS") to promises of amounts of weight loss over time periods that compute to rapid rates of weight loss. ("YOU CAN LOSE 18 POUNDS IN ONE WEEK!" "lose up to 10 lbs in 48 hours"). Additional examples are set forth in Table 4. Even the product names ("Redu-Quick, "Slim Down Fast") emphasize speedy results.

Such results are not only unlikely, they would be accomplished at an increased risk to health. Rapid weight loss has been associated with an increased risk of developing gallstones.[25] Consequently, responsible programs that offer proven means of rapid weight loss for obese patients with such diseases as coronary artery disease or Type II diabetes provide physician supervision while patients are actively losing weight.

Rapid weight-loss claims often appeared in combination with the promise of easy weight loss ("Lose those pounds the quick and easy way," "Lose weight while you sleep," "Lose weight quickly and easily and keep it off") without the need for diet or exercise. In 54% of the ads promising rapid weight loss, there are also claims for easy weight loss or weight loss without the need for changing diets or increasing exercise levels.

4. Lose Weight Without Diet or Exercise

Despite the well-accepted prescription of diet and exercise for successful weight management,26 42% of all of the ads reviewed promote a dizzying array of quick-fix pills, patches, potions, and programs for effortless weight loss. An ad for an apple cider vinegar pill, for example, boasts that "you can eat as much as you want and still lose weight," because "when properly distributed, an intake of 4,000 calories a day can actually help you lose weight instead of gain it." Another ad exclaims that a pill purportedly containing the "herbal equivalents" of ephedrine, caffeine, and aspirin, plus other ingredients, is "scientifically shown in a recent clinical study to elicit a 613% greater rate of fat loss in non-exercising subjects as compared to subjects not using it."[27] Additional examples are set forth in Table 5.[28]

In addition, 64% of the ads containing the effortless weight-loss claims outlined above also promise that the advertised products and services will produce fast results. These ads include such claims as "[t]ake off up to 10 pounds and 6" in just 2 days...[n]o exercise," "lose 3-4 pounds a week without dieting or exercise," "[I]'ve lost 68 lbs in 4 months...does not require restricted diets or exercise," and "[I] ate more and exercised less and still lost 44 lbs."

5. Lose Weight Permanently

"You lose it. You gain it back. Use [the advertised product] with every diet program and keep it off." Many consumers have lost weight only to gain it back again. In fact, studies indicate that most people who lose weight gain it back within five years.29 Consequently, "take it off and keep it off" claims are fairly common in weight-loss advertising. In spite of the blue-sky promises of many marketers ("Get weight off and keep it off," "You won't gain the weight back afterwards, because your weight will have reached its equilibrium," "Discover the secret to permanent weight loss"), experts have repeatedly observed that although persons generally lose weight while actively participating in a weight loss regimen treatment, they tend to regain the weight over time once treatment ends.30 According to the National Academy of Science Food and Nutrition Board, "Many programs and services exist to help individuals achieve weight control. But the limited studies paint a grim picture: those who complete weight-loss programs lose approximately 10 percent of their body weight only to regain two-thirds of it back within 1 year and almost all of it back within 5 years."31

For persons who have lost weight in the past only to gain it all back again, the appeal of a "once and forever" weight-loss product can be strong, especially when combined with references to the syndrome of failure many dieters experience or the promise of effortless, no-sacrifice weight-loss success. (Table 6) According to almost all weight-loss experts, if there is a key to long-term maintenance success, it requires permanent lifestyle changes on the part of the dieter: nutritional eating at moderate caloric levels, a regular physical fitness routine, and abandonment of old habits that may have contributed to weight gain.32

The publicly available scientific research contains very little evidence that would substantiate long-term or permanent weight-loss claims for most of today's popular diet products. Experts usually insist on studies going out at least one year, if not two, in order to substantiate a claim for long-term weight-loss maintenance.33 Reliable studies of the long-term effectiveness of weight-loss products and programs are difficult and expensive to conduct. Not many marketers are likely to want to spend the money and the time necessary to have such tests of their product's effectiveness done. But that does not prevent many of them from assuring consumers that their product or service is "the secret to permanent weight loss" or that "you may never need to diet again."

6. No Matter How Many Times You Failed Before

Among the weight-loss product advertisements surveyed, many contain "no more failure claims" that, although this may not be the first product tried, it will be the last. (Table 7) One marketer asks, for example: "Are you tired of fad diets that never seem to work? Are you frustrated when you gain back most or all of the weight you lose? Are you fed up with throwing money down the drain on diets that don't work?" This marketer, of course, claims to offer the one product that will finally work.

Many advertisers take an empathetic and understanding tone, assuring consumers that they are not to blame for their failure to lose weight:

Dear Friend: If you've ever tried losing weight using one of the hundred diets programs available, you know how difficult and frustrating it can be. And you are not alone. Most people who sincerely – even desperately – want to lose weight have never been successful on a diet. That's because diets do not work.

Others take advantage of the difficulty many consumers have in maintaining lost weight:

You've been there. You want to lose weight, and you've been successful before. But after a while, you're right back where you started - and the pounds always seem to come back . . . [The advertised product] can help you break the cycle.

This advertising technique frequently takes the form of a testimonial from a product user who confides that he or she has experienced the same weight-loss frustrations:

Discouraged, I started trying all the tricks, appetite suppressants, creams, diets and medications. Fads came and went and I had spent a fortune with no result. Of course, I tried to lose weight numerous times. But each new diet left me starved and deprived. I'd lose weight, but end up irritable and unhappy. Diets weakened me physically and emotionally. I once lost all my weight on a liquid fast. It was incredibly expensive. Of course, the weight came right back on.

As a result of extravagant advertising claims such as the ones described in this report, consumers may develop unrealistic notions about how much weight they can lose or keep off. Consumers purchase products purporting to be "unique" or "revolutionary" in their effectiveness and experience failure after failure.

7. Scientifically Proven/Doctor Endorsed

Many marketers attempt to bolster the credibility of their claims by asserting that the advertised product has been scientifically tested and proven to work. (Table 8) Phrases like "the clinically proven healthy way to lose weight," "clinically tested," "scientifically proven," and "studies confirm" bestow products with an aura of scientific legitimacy and aim to persuade consumers that they should feel confident that a product will work.

Several advertisements describe the dramatic results obtained in clinical studies. One advertisement, for example, asserts that "Clinical studies show people lost 300% more weight even without dieting."[34] Many advertisements also tout the fact that products were either developed or tested at well-known, respected, and "independent" institutions, such as "major universities," "a leading U.S. medical center," or "leading hospital[s]." Other advertisements showcase the impressive credentials of the researchers conducting the studies supporting the product, such as an advertisement that claims that a study proving the efficacy of the product was conducted by "the country's most respected scientists."

Many advertisers also imply that there is a substantial body of competently conducted scientific research supporting the efficacy of the product.[35] For instance, one advertisement claims that the efficacy of a product is "[b]acked by volumes of independent research and hundreds of published studies by the most prominent universities and medical journals in the world." Another marketer claims that "[s]cientists dedicated years of research to come up with a high powered diet ingredient [contained in the product] with no side effects."

Although some advertisements briefly describe the results, and provide some information about the methodology, of a particular study, such as the study's duration and number of participating subjects, most of the advertisements fail to give consumers sufficient detail about a study to allow consumers to verify the advertiser's representations. Moreover, 20 of the 117 ads making "clinically proven" claims were for products that contained ingredients already evaluated by the Federal Trade Commission in the context of past law enforcement actions challenging specific weight loss claims. These ingredients, which include fucus vesiculosus, chromium, L-carnitine, chitosan, psyllium, 7-keto-DHEA, hydroxycitric acid, seaweed, konjac root, garcinia cambogia and glucomannan, were challenged based on insufficient scientific evidence to support the weight loss claims made in the advertisements.

Still another technique that advertisers use to convince consumers that they are buying a tested and proven product is to assure consumers that a product is "recommended," "approved by," and often "developed" or "discovered" by a medical professional. (Table 8) For example, several advertisements prominently feature a "physician" wearing a white lab coat and a stethoscope and sitting in front of a diploma-filled wall. To add an air of legitimacy to the advertised product, some advertisements appear to be written by a physician. Others feature interviews with doctors or researchers who tout the product as being safe and effective. One Internet site even invites customers to call a "Medical Advisory Board" staffed with "qualified medical professionals" to answer medical questions.

Expert endorsements, however, can be misleading. For example, an advertisement may fail to disclose that the medical professional endorsing the product has a financial interest in promoting the sale of the product – a fact likely to affect the weight consumers give the endorsement and that could affect their purchase decision.[36] Marketers may even use a fictitious medical professional to endorse their products.[37] In other instances, experts either may not have actually reviewed the scientific evidence on the product or its ingredients or failed to utilize existing expert standards in conducting their review.[38]

8. Money-back Guarantees

The analysis revealed that money-back guarantees are one of the most frequently used techniques in weight-loss advertising. Fifty-two percent (52%) of all the ads reviewed include this representation. (Table 9) One advertiser, for example, encourages consumers to pay the price of the product only if the product has helped the consumer slim down: "If not, send it back and pay nothing. There will be no questions asked and you won't owe us a dime." Another advertiser advises consumers that the company would not guarantee its products if they did not work as advertised: "Believe me, I am not a gambler. I would never provide such an opportunity if I wasn't totally convinced that this is the weight-loss breakthrough of the decade, and there's no need to worry about too many requests for refunds."

Although many companies guarantee "consumer satisfaction" in general, several advertisements make very specific guarantees: "Whether you diet or not, [the marketer] guarantees that you'll lose up to seven pounds in the first week and then one dress or pant size every two weeks thereafter, or pay nothing." Another marketer promises consumers that, "no matter how many times you've tried before . . . no matter how much weight you have to lose . . . no matter how sluggish your metabolism . . . you will lose up to 10 to 15 pounds in just one week . . . up to 35 pounds in 3 weeks. Yes. Guaranteed! You lose or it doesn't cost you a penny."

For any number of reasons, marketers may fail to honor refund requests at all or delay honoring them for months. In fact, the Federal Trade Commission has brought several cases against marketers failing to make refunds promised in their advertising.[39]

9. Safe/All Natural Claims

Safety claims are a prevalent marketing technique in weight-loss advertising. Nearly half of all the ads in the sample (42%) contained specific claims that the advertised products or services are safe. These claims are made in a variety of ways. Some ads contain direct, unqualified representations about the safety of the product or service in producing weight loss, including such statements as "safe and effective," "100% safe and natural," "safe and gentle as a vitamin pill," "safe, immediate weight loss," and "safely lose up to 6 lbs of fat, fluid, and flesh in just the first 24 hours alone." Others make direct comparisons between the safety of the product or service and other weight-loss methods, with claims like "safer than liposuction," "safest and most effective strategy [for weight loss]," and "safest weight management system in the world." Finally, some safety claims are combined with compelling assertions of scientific proof of safety. Examples of those claims include such statements as "proven safe and effective," "proven 100% safe," and "tested for years and found to be very safe."

Many other weight-loss advertisements strongly imply that the product or service is safe because it has no side effects, is not a prescription weight-loss drug, or contains no potentially harmful stimulants. These representations include claims like "no side effects," "no dangerous pills or tablets to take," "[pills] do not pose a health hazard," "88% success rate with virtually no side effects," "in no way can [product X] harm your health," "no dangerous dehydration nor depression," "contains no stimulants that can harm the heart, increase blood pressure...," "skip risking your health [from prescription drugs]," and "none of the harmful side effects often associated with prescription diet products." One ad claimed that "the active compound has been recognized by the FDA as safe and effective for weight loss."

Claims of "all natural" often appear in conjunction with safety claims. Almost three quarters (71%) of those ads containing safety claims also had "natural" claims. These two claims appeared in 30% of all the ads that we reviewed, often in the same sentence. Examples of combined claims include "100% natural with no side effects," "all natural 100% safe," "lose weight naturally, safely," "100% natural so it's totally safe," and "lose weight in an easy way that is natural and that won't hurt your body." Overall, 44% of the ads that we reviewed. made some version of the "all natural" claim.

Safety claims sometimes appeared in ads promoting the product in a way that could create the potential for injury. For example, 73% of the ads in our sample that contained safety claims also represented that the product or service would produce "fast," "quick," or "immediate" results. If the product actually worked as quickly as advertised, it could produce potentially dangerous results, because rapid weight loss and safety are antagonistic goals. In fact, rapid weight loss, if not closely monitored by a physician, can result in serious adverse health consequences.[40]

Finally, of those weight-loss advertisements that contained safety claims, 27% also included some type of safety-related warning in the advertisements. These warnings varied widely in substance and detail. Some stated simply that you should "consult your doctor," or "consult your physician before beginning this or any weight-loss or exercise program." Others included more targeted warnings, such as "do not use this product if you have high blood pressure, are pregnant or breast feeding, or on medication for a heart condition." Often, the safety warning is presented in a manner that viewers are likely not to notice it.

One ad contained a warning about serious health effects: "[t]his product has ephedrine group alkaloids in the form of herbal extracts and may cause serious adverse health effects." This ad also included the claim that the product was "shown to be safe by two independent laboratories." Conflicting messages in an advertisement about safety may confuse consumers and, ultimately, may cause them to ignore safety-related warnings.

Safety claims for weight-loss products are of serious concern. The primary concern is that potentially serious adverse health effects can result if the claim is untrue or the effects of a product are unproven. This concern is particularly important where the product may present special undisclosed risks for certain populations, such as pregnant women or nursing mothers, or where the long-term health effects are unknown. In addition, certain products or ingredients may interact adversely with other medications that consumers might be taking, or may exacerbate pre-existing health conditions faced by overweight and obese consumers, including, for example, heart disease, high blood pressure, and diabetes. Ephedra or ephedrine alkaloids, for example, may be associated with dangerous effects on the central nervous system and heart and may result in serious injury for some persons.[41]

Almost half (48%) of the ads that identified ephedra as a product ingredient made safety claims, yet only slightly more than half of those (55%) included a specific warning about the health risks of ephedra. Only 30% of all ads that identified ephedra as an ingredient included a specific health warning about its potential adverse effects. Even more disturbing from a safety perspective, fully 60% of ads that made safety claims did not identify ingredients at all. Consumers' inability to make informed decisions about the safety of such products clearly raises the potential for serious adverse health consequences.

VI. Media Responsibility

Advertisements for weight-loss products and services too frequently contain extravagant and sensational efficacy claims that are scientifically groundless. Although many of them could be screened out by responsible media before they reach the public, mainstream newspapers, magazines, radio stations, and broadcast and cable TV outlets run ads for weight-loss products that strain credibility. Moreover, the appearance of these ads in what appear to be reputable publications may increase the credibility of the promotions and serve to overcome or reduce consumer skepticism. This problem may be exacerbated in the case of publications that consumers purchase, such as newspapers, if consumers view these publications to be sources of more credible information than advertisements that are essentially free to consumers, e.g., direct mail solicitations. It is apparent that most media make little or no attempt to screen questionable ads for weight-loss products. The major televison broadcast networks, ABC, CBS, and NBC, are an exception. These networks employ stringent advertising clearance standards that require advertisers to submit proposed advertisements, along with adequate substantiation for all claims, to the networks for review prior to dissemination. As an illustration, with regard to weight reduction and control products, ABC's published standards prohibit, among other practices, unsubstantiated claims and representations that weight loss is simple, quick, or easy.[86] There are other exceptions as well. For example, *Good Housekeeping Magazine* has a policy of not running any advertisements containing facially false or dubious weight loss claims.

Recent efforts to heighten media awareness have been largely unsuccessful. In May 2000, The Partnership for Healthy Weight Management inaugurated a campaign to promote media responsibility for the weight-loss advertising publishers disseminate. *Ad Nauseam*, as the initiative was named, sought to call the media's attention to the many groundless claims appearing in ads they publish. Claims that the Partnership identified include the following:

- Lose up to 2 Pounds Daily . . . Without Diet or Exercise
- Imagine Losing As Much As 50% Of All Excess Fat In Just 14 Days! Not Even Total Starvation Can Slim You down and Firm You up this Fast - this Safely! . . . Lose up to 1 Full Pound Every 8 Hours. Lose up to 2 1/2 to 3 Full Pounds Each Day and you do it without counting calories.
- U.S. Patent reveals weight loss of as much as 28 lbs. in 4 weeks and 48 lbs. in 8 weeks.... Eat all your favorite foods and still lose weight (pill does all the work).
- New Medical Breakthrough! Lose A Pound A Day Without Changing What You Eat. No impossible exercise! No missed meals! No dangerous pills. No boring foods or small portions!"
- You lose weight even if you eat too much.... You will lose at least 16 pounds in the first two weeks. And at least six pounds every week thereafter.

These claims and other similar claims cited in the Ad Nauseam campaign appeared in such publications as *Cosmopolitan, Esquire, McCall's, Redbook, Woman's Day, The*

Laura Muha

Atlanta Journal - Constitution, *The [Denver] Rocky Mountain News*, *USA Today*, and *Smart Source* (a publication of News America, FSI, Inc.). Unfortunately, the media, for the most part, have failed to respond to the Partnership's message. As reflected in this report, and as the examples set forth in Appendix B illustrate, ads for weight-loss products promising dubious outcomes still appear regularly in mainstream media. Table 11 provides a list of the top 30 magazines and tabloids that published ads collected for this report. In most instances, a single ad appeared in more than one publication.

Most broadcasters and publishers already screen ads for taste and appropriateness, but too often the screening process stops short of questioning the accuracy of facially extravagant claims. As this report demonstrates, this shortcoming is particularly apparent in the area of ads for weight-loss products and services. Fraudulent ads cost legitimate advertisers and consumers millions of dollars each year. Government agencies and self-regulatory groups can step in once the ad has been disseminated to an unwary public, but only the media can stop false ads before they are disseminated.

Effective ad clearance standards reduce the damaging effects of advertising fraud on American consumers and commerce. Exercising responsibility in the screening of advertising for weight-loss products and services is a way that the media can contribute to the Surgeon General's Call to Action to Prevent and Decrease Overweight and Obesity 2001. That document characterized the media's role in the following manner:

> The media can provide essential functions in overweight and obesity prevention efforts. From a public education and social marketing standpoint, the media can disseminate health messages and display healthy behaviors aimed at changing dietary habits and exercise patterns.[87]

Among the strategies that the Call to Action recommended for the media was to "[e]ncourage truthful and reasonable consumer goals for weight-loss programs and weight management products."[88] This report underscores that in responding to the Surgeon General's Call to Action, the media must assess not only how their editorial content can meet the challenge, but most importantly, how their revenue generating divisions can respond to the call and "promote truthful and reasonable consumer goals" through the advertising they accept.

VII. Conclusion

False promises of effortless weight loss feed on and exacerbate consumers' hunger for the easy fix to overweight and obesity. Consumers taken in by such attractive claims lose both economically, by wasting resources on products that do not work as advertised, and medically, by foregoing or postponing other weight-loss methods and necessary lifestyle changes that have demonstrated benefits in reducing the adverse health consequences of overweight and obesity.

The use of deceptive and misleading claims in weight-loss advertising is rampant. Nearly 40% of the ads in our sample made at least one representation that almost certainly is false. The vast majority of these ads were for dietary supplements or hypnosis. In addition, 55% of the ads in our sample made at least one representation that is very likely to be false or, at the very least, lacks adequate substantiation. Some of the more obvious questionable representations include:

- Specific performance claims, such as lose up to 10 pounds per week, that are outside the realm of possibility for the products being advertised;
- Claims that users can lose substantial amounts of weight rapidly without diet or exercise;
- Testimonials claiming weight loss that exceed what is physiologically possible under normal circumstances, for example, losing 120 pounds in seven weeks;
- Claims that weight loss will be long-term or permanent; and
- Unqualified safety claims or confusing representations concerning safety for ingredients known to have

Laura Muha

potential risks for a significant number of users or to have potential adverse interactions with commonly prescribed prescription drugs.

Below this level, a considerable number of advertisements contain claims that may be misleading or unsubstantiated. Determining whether the claims in this category are actually deceptive would require further inquiry, such as reviewing the substantiation the advertiser has to support the claim.

The proliferation of misleading weight-loss ads has proceeded in the face of, and in spite of, an unprecedented level of FTC enforcement. Although conclusive evidence is not available, what evidence there is suggests that the incidence of false and deceptive claims has increased over the last decade. It is beyond the scope of this report to recommend specific remedies to combat this growing problem. Nevertheless, the need for critical evaluation seems readily apparent. Government agencies with oversight over weight-loss advertising must continually reassess the effectiveness of enforcement and consumer and business education strategies. Critical questions include whether the level of resources currently devoted to law enforcement is adequate; whether more specific advice to advertisers would improve compliance; and if so, how to provide that advice.

Trade associations and self-regulatory groups must do a better job of educating their members about fair advertising standards and enforcing those standards. This is a particularly difficult challenge. Even companies that subscribe to a self-regulatory code may feel competitive pressure to exaggerate their claims in the face of a marketplace that seems out of control. Unless self-regulatory groups are willing to review questionable advertisements, take disciplinary action where appropriate, and publicize their decisions, the industry as a whole will continue to suffer from a lack of credibility. Even so, a significant amount of the questionable advertising identified in this report was generated by companies that are outside the mainstream of current self-regulatory efforts. With regard to these companies, selfregulation will have little, if any, effect.

It is clear from this report that false and misleading weight loss advertising is not limited to the back of supermarket tabloids. Many of the ads we identified as making almost certainly false claims appeared in mainstream media publications such as *Family Circle*, *Cosmopolitan*, *Women's Day*, *McCall's*, and *Redbook*. Although 74% of the ads in tabloid publications included at least one almost certainly false claim, so did 54% of the ads in newspapers and FSIs. The media must be encouraged to adopt clearance standards that weed out facially deceptive and misleading weight-loss claims. In most cases, the questionable claims arc not hard to identify and asking advertisers for substantiation is not unreasonable. Improved lines of communications between government and self-regulatory groups and publishers could also be beneficial. Although the ultimate decision of whether to disseminate a particular advertisement rests with the publisher, improved communications could be useful in alerting publishers to ads and claims that pose problems.

Finally, individual consumers must become more knowledgeable about the importance of achieving and maintaining healthy weight, more informed about how to shop for weight-loss products and services, and more skeptical of ads promising quick-fixes. Government and industry share a responsibility to insure that accurate and understandable information about weight loss treatments is readily available to consumers. As one expert notes, success will come when the public is convinced "that there is no 'magic bullet.'"[89]

Appendix A

Product List

3 Day Diet Plan
48 Hour cyclone diet
A Nu You
ABC Diet Program
Advanced Weight Loss
Advanced Weight Loss &
    Wellness
AdvantRx Weight Loss
    Accelerator
Advocare
Algoxyll
Alph-Lean
AM-300
Amazing Mega Trim
Amerifit Fatburner System
Ann Morgan Book
Anorex
Aoqili Premium Seaweed Soap
Apidex-P
Apple Cider Vinegar Capsules
Aprinol
AS-200
Asparagus Superactivated
    Tablets
Atkins Diet
Banish Your Belly, Butt and
    Thighs Forever
Bariatric Treatment Centers
Berry Trim Plus

BeTrimToo's Liquid Drops
BeeTrimToo's Thin
Beverly Hills Fat Burners
BioGenesis
BioSculpt
Blast Away Fat
Body Furnace
Body Type Supplement
Botanic Choice Apple Cider
    Vinegar
Calorad
Calorad 2000
Caloslim 2000
Calotrol/M.D.
Caltrim
Carb Cutter
Carb Trapper Plus
Carb Fighter
Callucal
CalluLife Anti-cellulite Fashion
    Hosiery
Cellulite Reduction Cream
CelluRid
Changes Now Super Fat
    Binder
Cheat and Lean
Chito-Trim
Chitogenics
Chitosan

Chitosol
ChromasTherm
Cutting Gel
Cyclone Diet System
Cytodyne Xenadrine
Cytoplex
Dallas Hypnosis Center
Dermalin-Apg
Dessert Avert
DetoX
Didrex
dietdivas
DietMagic
DietSmart
Doctor's Fat Burner
DoctorsCare
Dr. Sandra Cabot's Natural
    Health Formulas
Dr. Jackish's Redu-Quick
Dynamic Fatburner
EAS Betalean
Exercise in a Bottle
Extreme Power Plus
Fast-Burn
Fat-B-Gone
Fat Complexer
Fat Fighter
Fat Metabolizer Capsules
Fat Neutralizer
Fat-Sponge in a Pill
Fat Trapper Plus
Fit America
Forever Young (HGH)
Fostec
Friendly 7
Gentle Ferocity

Get Slim Slippers
Goen Method
Gorayeb Weightloss Seminar
Grow.Lean 15
Herbal Body Wrap
High Protein Low-Carb Diet
    Quick Weight Loss Diet
Hollywood 48-Hour Miracle Diet
Human Growth Hormone
Hunger Ease
Hydroxycut
Inches-A-Weigh
Inferno
Ionamin
Jenny Craig
Kaloski Method
KarbKiller
Kashi Cereals
LA Weight Loss Centers
Lipordrene
Lipoguard
LipoSlim
Lipotrophic Injections
Livatone
LivLite Weight Management
    Program
Luprinol
Magic Herb Diet Plus
    Chromium Picolinate
Mega Apple Cider Plus
Meridia
Meta-Biological Dietary
    Supplement
Metabolic Weight Loss Center
Metabolic Research Center
Metabolic Thyrolean

Metabolic Weight Loss
Metabolife (shakes, diet and energy bars)
Metabolife 356
Metabolift
MeTrim Block
MeTrim Night
MeTrim SuperBlock
Miami 48 Hour Diet
Millenium Diet
Miracle Diet Formula
Nature's Shape
Negative Calorie Diet ebook
newStart
Nu Life
Nutri/System
Oleda Super Fat Burner
OptiBurn
Optifast
Optifast Plan
Oral GH formula
Oxycise
OZ Garcia's Celebrity Slim 5 Day Diet Plan
PatentLEAN
Phentermine
Physicians Weight Loss Centers
Picture Perfect Weight Loss
Plant Macerat
Positive Changes Hypnosis Centers
Power Diet Plus
Prescriptions for Healthy Living
Protein and Plus Diet System

Pure Lipotric Fat-Burner Tablets
Quick Slim
redu-quick
Richard Simmons' Lose Weight and Celebrate Plan
RS-Fire
Satietrol
Scan Diet
Sea Clay Body Wrap
Serotril
Shipula Center Hypnosis
Simply Slender Body Wraps
Simply Slym
Skinny Me
Sleep A Weigh
Slender Life Weight Loss Centers
Slender Now Weight Management Program
Slenderstrip
Slendior
Slimdown Fast
SlimSense System
Stay-N-Thin Rapid Burn Diet
Suddenly Slender
Super Fat Burner System
Super Shaper 2000
Synadrene-HCL
Synergie Lifestyle System
TG-2000 Fat Burner
The Body Wrap
The Original Hollywood Celebrity Diet
The Ultimate Weight Loss eBook

Thermal Carb
Thermo Balance
Thermo Life
Thermo-Lift Classic
Thermo-Lift II
Thermo-Lift
Thermo Phen Fen
Thermogencis Plus Stimulant
  Free
ThermoGencis Plus Quick
  Start
ThermoGold
Thermojetics Weight-
  Management Program
ThermoSlim
ThermoSulp
Thyro-Slim A.M./P.M.
ThyroStart
Thyrox T-3
Tonalin CLA
ToppFast
Tri-Amacil
Trim Spa
Trimlife
TrimSpa
Triphetamine
Twin Lab CLA Fuel
U.S. Women's Alpine Ski
  Team Diet
Ultra Carbo Block 2000
Ultra Carbohydrate Blocker
  2000
Ultra Slim-Fast
Ultra Trim 2000
Vinegar Weightloss Plan
Vita-Green

Bitala Trim
Weight Watchers
Xenadrine RFA-1
Xenical
Xeta Lean
Zymax

Notes

Introduction

". . . have beneficial changes to your cholesterol profile." (Interview with William Yancy, 2004)

". . . that doesn't mean it's good for you." (Interview with Dean Ornish, 2000)

". . . 'the grease Gestapo." (*Los Angeles Times*, 7/26/04)

". . . the vegetarian Taliban." (*Dateline NBC*, 2/20/04)

". . . why, why, why?" (http://forum.lowcarber.org/archive/index.php/t-208432.html)

". . . I had to spit it into my napkin." (*New York Daily News*, 1/21/04)

". . . nutrition issues surrounding bread. (http://www.breadcouncil.org/NBLC_site_11_07_03.swf)

". . . dismiss very-low-carbohydrate diets." (*Annals of Internal Medicine*, May 2004)

". . . the people who write popular diet books." (Interview with Walter Willett, 2004)

". . . there might be significant risk." (Interview with Diane Stadler, 2004)

". . . what we believe will happen." (Interview with William Yancy, 2004)

Chapter 1: Low-Carb vs. Low-Fat: The Battle Begins

". . . I have three chins!'" (Interview with Robert Atkins, 2000)

". . . as mainstream as you could be." (Interview with Robert Atkins, 2000)

". . . skinniest kid on the block." (*Dr. Atkins' Diet Revolution*, p. 21)

". . . no one's going to be interested in me!'" (Interview with Robert Atkins, 2000)

". . . one hell of an appetite." (Interview with Robert Atkins, 2000)

". . . a low-calorie diet for even one day." (*Dr. Atkins' Diet Revolution*, p. 22)

". . . what I could do for myself." (*Dr. Atkins' Diet Revolution*, p. 23)

". . . I wanted to know why." (*Dr. Atkins' Diet Revolution*, p. 23)

". . . and loss of appetite." (http://www.usda.gov/cnpp/Seminars/GND/Proceedings.txt)

". . . diet I've ever been on." (http://www.usda.gov/cnpp/Seminars/GND/Proceedings.txt)

". . . still lose, without hunger." (*Dr. Atkins' Diet Revolution*, p. 25)

". . . the more you lost." (Interview with Robert Atkins, 2000)

". . . hadn't been feeling up to par." (*Dr. Atkins' Diet Revolution*, p. 27)

". . . the first time playing golf!" (Interview with Robert Atkins, 2000)

". . . potentially dangerous."(*Reason*, March 2003)

". . . life has been dedicated to that." (Interview with Robert Atkins, 2000)

". . . a long list of harmful foods. (http://www.cdc.gov/mmwr/preview/mmwrhtml/mm4830a1box.htm)

". . . will reduce saturated fat intake." (*Food Politics*, p. 42)

". . . ever had, and it's failed." (Interview with Michael Eades, 2004)

". . . exploited for commercial benefit." (Interview with Ruth Kava, 2004)

" . . . which was insanity." (Interview with Linda Stern, 2004)

" . . . decreasing the numerator." (Interview with Ruth Kava, 2004)

" . . . the salad, the leafy vegetables?" (*The Physiology of Taste*, p.251)

" . . . season is over." (http://www.lowcarbing.com/downloads/banting.pdf)

" . . . flabby and baggy." (*Near a Thousand Tables: A History of Food*, p. 47)

" . . . into cakes and broiled." (*Near a Thousand Tables: A History of Food*, p. 47)

" . . . protein, carbs, and fats."(http://www.drsears.com/drsearspages/zonemondaypage.jsp)

Chapter 2: An Introduction to Metabolism

"...up talking about the same thing." (Interview with Linda Stern, 2004)

" . . . more protein as well." (Interview with Walter Willett, 2004)

" . . .to make carbohydrates out of that." (Interview with Joanne Lupton, 2004)

" . . . effect on the body." (Interview with Eric Westman, 2004)

" . . . makes fat look good!" (Interview with Joanne Lupton, 2004)

" . . . just in the first few days." (Interview with Joanne Lupton, 2004)

" . . . drawbacks than either of them." (*Dr. Atkins' New Diet Revolution*, 1992 ed., p. 52)

" . . . starving to death." (Interview with Marion Nestle, 2004)

" . . . they do what they want." (Interview with Diane Stadler, 2004)

Chapter 3: Weighty Issues: Do You Really Lose More on a Low-Carb Diet?

" . . . to keep me motivated." (Interview with Jaynelle Tenor, 2004)

". . . never happened for me." (Interview with Bill Tenor, 2004)

". . . work-in-all-circumstances statements." (*Protein Power*, p. XV)

". . . controlled carbohydrate nutritional approach." (*Dr. Atkins New Diet Revolution*, 2002 ed., p. 64)

". . . at 300 to 400 calories a day." (Interview with Michael Eades, 2004)

". . . true in the longer-duration studies." (Interview with William Yancy, 2004)

". . . they just weren't hungry." (Interview with Eric Westman, 2004)

". . . tightly controlled study." (Interview with Diane Stadler, 2004)

". . . that's really impressive." (Interview with Diane Stadler, 2004)

". . . for a conventional healthy diet." (Interview with Diane Stadler, 2004)

". . . that was our bottom line." (Interview with Diane Stadler, 2004)

". . . just not in my schedule." (Interview with Jaynelle Tenor, 2004)

". . . affecting our diet in some ways." (Interview with Jaynelle Tenor, 2004)

". . . not the right diet for me." (Interview with Bill Tenor, 2004)

Chapter 4: The Heart of the Matter

". . . would be pulled off the market." (Interview with Neal Barnard, 2004)

". . . saturated fat can trigger a heart attack!" (*The South Beach Diet*, p. 22)

". . . you do dramatically better." (*Today*, 2000)

". . . lipid issue is really complex." (Interview with Michael Eades, 2004)

". . . wouldn't have normal cholesterol." (Interview with

Michael Eades, 2004)

". . . not insignificant." (Interview with Diane Stadler, 2004)

". . . them on appropriate medications." (Interview with Diane Stadler, 2004)

". . . what happens beyond that." (Interview with Samuel Klein, 2004)

". . . effectiveness of this approach." (Interview with Samuel Klein, 2004)

". . . falls into this category." (*Dr. Atkins' New Diet Revolution*, 1992 ed., p. 145)

". . . diet that you enjoyed more." (*Dr. Atkins' New Diet Revolution*, 1992 ed., p. 146)

". . . does he say to get off the diet." (Interview with Jody Gorran, 2004)

". . . absence of refined carbohydrates." (http://atkins.com/Archive/2001/12/18-292461.html)

". . . something that nobody else knew." (Interview with Jody Gorran, 2004)

". . . would listen how great it was." (Interview with Jody Gorran, 2004)

". . . I wasn't really worried." (Interview with Jody Gorran, 2004)

". . . on the low-carb diet." (Interview with Jody Gorran, 2004)

". . . the minute I got in the cab." (Interview with Jody Gorran, 2004)

". . . pushing on my heart." (Interview with Jody Gorran, 2004)

". . .was misled and betrayed." (Interview with Jody Gorran, 2004)

". . . I'd never eaten before." (Interview with Jody Gorran, 2004)

". . . It's unethical." (Interview with Jody Gorran, 2004)

". . . medicine that affects change." (Interview with Stuart L. Trager, 2004)

". . . frivolous ... distraction." (Interview with Stuart L. Trager, 2004)

". . . a horrible group." (Interview with Stuart L. Trager, 2004)

". . . goal is to sell things." (Interview with Neal Barnard, 2004)

"... have them singing 'Kumbaya.'" (Interview with Neal Barnard, 2004)

"... as evidence of wrongdoing." (http://atkins.com/Archive/2004/5/28-354036.html)

"... if they are operative for you." (*Dr. Atkins' New Diet Revolution*, 1992 ed., p. 145)

"... fat-restricted variation of the diet." (*Dr. Atkins' New Diet Revolution*, 1992 ed., p. 146)

"... helped by this [low-carb] approach." (Interview with Stuart L. Trager, 2004)

"... something like that, I'd consider it." (Interview with Jody Gorran, 2004)

"... bad for your arteries, Bill."(http://www.nealhendrickson.com/mcdougall/2004lbn/040904news.htm)

"... to diminish heart disease. (http://cnnstudentnews.cnn.com/TRANSCRIPTS/0409/06/ltm.02.html)

"... well as diet and exercise."(http://cnnstudentnews.cnn.com/TRANSCRIPTS/0409/06/ltm.02.html)

"... tell us what was wrong." (Interview with Paul Huskey, 2004)

"... body's potential response to it." (*Southern Medical Journal*, Sept. 1, 2002)

"... abnormality like that." (Interview with Stuart Trager, 2004)

"... She was never sick." (Interview with Paul Huskey, 2004)

"... risks are before you start." (Interview with Paul Huskey, 2004)

Chapter 5: The Long-Term Effects

"... do long term that is of relevance." (Interview with Suzanne Havala-Hobbs, 2004)

"... price we're going to pay." (Interview with Barbara Moore, 2004)

"... obesity and overweight." (Interview with Colette Heimowitz, 2004)

"...''It's a tool." (Interview with Colette Heimowitz, 2004)

"... like you do with cancer." (Interview with Walter Willett, 2004)

"... significant increase in urinary calcium." (*The American Journal of Medicine, Vol. 113*, p.33)

"... you eat a diet like that." (Interview with Michael Eades, 2004)

"... I believe you'll be fine." (Interview with Michael Eades, 2004)

"... careful about a high-protein diet." (Interview with Ellie Schlam, 2004)

"... not the supplement." (Interview with Joanne Lupton, 2004)

"... of normal tissue function." (*The Medical Journal Of Australia (1977):65*)

"... on the dietary regime." (*The Medical Journal Of Australia (1977):65*)

"... I'm going to die." (Interview with Mary Madlem, 2004)

"... just didn't work at all." (Interview with Mary Madlem, 2004)

Chapter 6: The Business of Low-Carb

"... make weight management easier."(http://www.usatoday.com/money/industries/food/2004-09-26-kraft-usat_x.htm)

"... sabotage low-carb diets." (Interview with Linda Stern 2004)

"... they were already eating?" (Interview with Linda Stern 2004)

"... low-fat. We can't be a fad." (http://www.lowcarbiz.com/public/198.cfm)

"... help anybody lose weight." (Interview with Marion Nestle, 2004)

"... marketing them as low-carb." (Interview with Suzanne Prong Eygabroat, 2004)

"... that give people diarrhea." (Interview with Colette Heimowitz, 2004)

"... science of marketing low carb." (Interview with Suzanne Prong Eygabroat, 2004)

Laura Muha

"... to help dieters succeed." (Interview with Colette Heimowitz, 2004)

"... right thing is helping people." (Interview with Stuart L. Trager, 2004)

"... but don't get results." (Interview with Stuart L. Trager, 2004)

"... going to work with kids?" (Interview with Keith-Thomas Ayoob, 2004)

"... information at vulnerable children."(http://www.wate.com/Global/story.asp?S=2360007)

"... saying 'How can we help?'" (Interview with Stuart L. Trager, 2004)

"... our kids for financial gain." (Interview with Keith-Thomas Ayoob, 2004)

"... do what we can to help." (Interview with Stuart L. Trager, 2004)

"... products out fast enough." (Interview with Suzanne Prong Eygabroat, 2004)

"... for quite a long time." (Interview with Suzanne Prong Eygabroat, 2004)

"... knock it off its pedestal." (Interview with Suzanne Prong Eygabroat, 2004)

Chapter 7: Is Low-Carb the Right Approach for You?

"... the best way to do it." (Interview with Eric Westman, 2004)

"... stick to in the long run." (Interview with Walter Willett, 2004)

"... under a doctor's supervision." (Interview with Eric Westman, 2004)

"... that can be dangerous." (Interview with William Yancy, 2004)

"... change your body metabolism." (Interview with Eric Westman, 2004)

"... actually pretty good." (Interview with Walter Willett, 2004)

"... a little more slowly." (Interview with Walter Willett, 2004)

"... with for the long run." (Interview with Walter Willett, 2004)

182

"... diet should consider this." (Interview with Samuel Klein, 2004)

"... eat the better off you are." (Interview with Michael Eades, 2004)

"... and measure everything." (Interview with Eric Westman, 2004)

"...the safety of the diet." (Interview with Eric Westman, 2004)

"... really the doctor's judgment." (Interview with Eric Westman, 2004)